Community Mental Health

DATE DUE			
21/5/19			

Other recent World Psychiatric Association titles

Special Populations

The Mental Health of Children and Adolescents: an area of global neglect
Edited by Helmut Remschmidt, Barry Nurcombe, Myron L. Belfer, Norman Sartorius and Ahmed Okasha
ISBN: 9780470512456

Contemporary Topics in Women's Mental Health: global perspectives in a changing society
Edited by Prabha S. Chandra, Helen Herrman, Marianne Kastrup, Marta Rondon, Unaiza Niaz, Ahmed Okasha, Jane Fisher
ISBN: 9780470754115

Parenthood and Mental Health: A bridge between infant and adult psychiatry
Edited by Sam Tyano, Miri Keren, Helen Herrman and John Cox
ISBN: 978-0-470-74722-3

Approaches to Practice and Research

Religion and Psychiatry: beyond boundaries
Edited by Peter J Verhagen, Herman M van Praag, Juan José López-Ibor, John Cox, Driss Moussaoui
ISBN: 9780470694718

Psychiatric Diagnosis: challenges and prospects
Edited by Ihsan M. Salloum and Juan E. Mezzich
ISBN: 9780470725696

Recovery in Mental Health: reshaping scientific and clinical responsibilities
By Michaela Amering and Margit Schmolke
ISBN: 9780470997963

Handbook of Service User Involvement in Mental Health Research
Edited by Jan Wallcraft, Beate Schrank and Michaela Amering
ISBN: 9780470997956

Psychiatrists and Traditional Healers: unwitting partners in global mental health
Edited by Mario Incayawar, Ronald Wintrob and Lise Bouchard,
ISBN: 9780470516836

Depression and Comorbidity

Depression and Diabetes
Edited by Wayne Katon, Mario Maj and Norman Sartorius
ISBN: 9780470688380

Depression and Heart Disease
Edited by Alexander Glassman, Mario Maj and Norman Sartorius
ISBN: 9780470710579

Depression and Cancer
Edited by David W. Kissane, Mario Maj and Norman Sartorius
ISBN: 9780470689660

World Psychiatric Association *Evidence and Experience in Psychiatry* Series

Series Editor: Helen Herrman, WPA Secretary for Publications, University of Melbourne, Australia

Post-traumatic Stress Disorder
Edited by Dan J. Stein, Matthew Friedman and Carlos Blanco
ISBN: 9780470688977

Depressive Disorders, 3e
Edited by Helen Herrman, Mario Maj and Norman Sartorius
ISBN: 9780470987209

Substance Abuse Disorders
Edited by Hamid Ghodse, Helen Herrman, Mario Maj and Norman Sartorius
ISBN: 9780470745106

Schizophrenia 2e
Edited by Mario Maj, Norman Sartorius
ISBN: 9780470849644

Dementia 2e
Edited by Mario Maj, Norman Sartorius
ISBN: 9780470849637

Obsessive-Compulsive Disorders 2e
Edited by Mario Maj, Norman Sartorius, Ahmed Okasha, Joseph Zohar
ISBN: 9780470849668

Bipolar Disorders
Edited by Mario Maj, Hagop S Akiskal, Juan José López-Ibor, Norman Sartorius
ISBN: 9780471560371

Eating Disorders
Edited by Mario Maj, Kathrine Halmi, Juan José López-Ibor, Norman Sartorius
ISBN: 9780470848654

Phobias
Edited by Mario Maj, Hagop S Akiskal, Juan José López-Ibor, Ahmed Okasha
ISBN: 9780470858332

Personality Disorders
Edited by Mario Maj, Hagop S Akiskal, Juan E Mezzich
ISBN: 9780470090367

Somatoform Disorders
Edited by Mario Maj, Hagop S Akiskal, Juan E Mezzich, Ahmed Okasha
ISBN: 9780470016121

Community Mental Health

Putting policy into practice globally

Graham Thornicroft and Maya Semrau

Health Service and Population Research Department, Institute of Psychiatry,
King's College London, London, UK

Atalay Alem

Department of Psychiatry, Faculty of Medicine, Addis Ababa University, Addis Ababa, Ethiopia

Robert E. Drake

Dartmouth Medical School, Lebanon, USA

Hiroto Ito

National Institute of Mental Health, National Centre of Neurology and Psychiatry, Tokyo, Japan

Jair Mari

Department of Psychiatry, Universidade Federal de São Paulo, Brazil

Peter McGeorge

Urban Mental Health Research Institute, Inner City Health Program, St Vincent's Hospital,
Sydney, Australia

R. Thara

Schizophrenia Research Foundation (SCARF), Chennai, India

WILEY-BLACKWELL

A John Wiley & Sons, Ltd., Publication

This edition first published 2011, © 2011 by John Wiley & Sons, Ltd.

Wiley-Blackwell is an imprint of John Wiley & Sons, formed by the merger of Wiley's global Scientific, Technical and Medical business with Blackwell Publishing.

Registered Office
John Wiley & Sons, Ltd, The Atrium, Southern Gate, Chichester, West Sussex, PO19 8SQ, UK

Editorial Offices
9600 Garsington Road, Oxford, OX4 2DQ, UK
The Atrium, Southern Gate, Chichester, West Sussex, PO19 8SQ, UK
111 River Street, Hoboken, NJ 07030-5774, USA

For details of our global editorial offices, for customer services and for information about how to apply for permission to reuse the copyright material in this book please see our website at www.wiley.com/wiley-blackwell.

The right of the author to be identified as the author of this work has been asserted in accordance with the UK Copyright, Designs and Patents Act 1988.

Library of Congress Cataloging-in-Publication Data

Global mental health : putting community care into practice / Graham Thornicroft . . . [et al.].
    p. ; cm.
  Includes bibliographical references and index.
  ISBN 978-1-119-99865-5 (pbk.)
 1. Community mental health services.   2. World health.   I. Thornicroft, Graham.
  [DNLM: 1. Community Mental Health Services.   2. Health Policy.   3. Mental Disorders.
4. Mental Health.   5. World Health. WM   30.6]
  RA790.5.G55 2011
  362.196'89—dc23
                                                                    2011023058

A catalogue record for this book is available from the British Library.

This book is published in the following electronic formats: ePDF: 9781119979210; Wiley Online Library: 9781119979203; ePub: 9781119952145; Mobi: 9781119952152

Set in 9.5/13pt Meridien by Aptara Inc., New Delhi, India
Printed in Singapore by Ho Printing Singapore Pte Ltd

First Impression   2011

Contents

List of Contributors

Africa
Atalay Alem
Department of Psychiatry, Faculty of Medicine
Addis Ababa University
Addis Ababa
Ethiopia

Charlotte Hanlon
Department of Psychiatry, Faculty of Medicine
Addis Ababa University
Addis Ababa
Ethiopia

Dawit Wondimagegn
Department of Psychiatry, Faculty of Medicine
Addis Ababa University
Addis Ababa
Ethiopia

Australasia and South Pacific
Peter McGeorge
New Zealand Mental Health Commission
Thorndon
Wellington
New Zealand

Europe
Elizabeth Barley
Health Service and Population Research Department
Institute of Psychiatry
King's College London
London
UK

Ann Law
Health Service and Population Research Department
Institute of Psychiatry
King's College London
London
UK

Maya Semrau
Health Service and Population Research Department
Institute of Psychiatry
King's College London
London
UK

Graham Thornicroft
Health Service and Population Research Department
Institute of Psychiatry
King's College London
London
UK

North America
Robert E. Drake
Dartmouth Medical School
Lebanon, NH
USA

Eric Latimer
Douglas Hospital, Psychiatry Department
McGill University
Montreal, QC
Canada

Latin America and Caribbean
Renato Antunes Dos Santos
Department of Psychiatry
Universidade Federal de São Paulo
São Paulo
Brazil

Guilherme Gregorio
Department of Psychiatry
Universidade Federal de São Paulo
São Paulo
Brazil

Jair Mari
Department of Psychiatry
Universidade Federal de São Paulo
São Paulo
Brazil

Denise Razzouk
Department of Psychiatry
Universidade Federal de São Paulo
São Paulo
Brazil

South Asia
R. Padmavati
Schizophrenia Research Foundation (SCARF)
Chennai
Tamil Nadu
India

R. Thara
Schizophrenia Research Foundation (SCARF)
Chennai
Tamil Nadu
India

East and South-East Asia
Hiroto Ito
National Institute of Mental Health
National Centre of Neurology and Psychiatry
Tokyo
Japan

Yutaro Setoya
National Institute of Mental Health
National Centre of Neurology and Psychiatry
Tokyo
Japan

Yuriko Suzuki
National Institute of Mental Health
National Centre of Neurology and Psychiatry
Tokyo
Japan

Foreword

The development of community mental health care is currently ongoing, or at least planned, in many countries worldwide. The World Psychiatric Association (WPA) supports this process, aimed at allowing persons with mental disorders to have services available as close as possible to their locality, to be treated in the least restrictive environment, and to maintain their links within the community. We expect the implementation of community mental health care to improve patients' clinical outcomes, subjective quality of life, and satisfaction with care.

Experience has shown that the steps to be followed, the obstacles to be removed, and the mistakes to be avoided in the implementation of community mental health care are remarkably similar worldwide. The WPA decided therefore to establish a task force with the mandate to produce guidance on those issues, intended for psychiatrists, other mental health professionals, and policy makers of all countries of the world. This task force, led by Graham Thornicroft and including experts from all continents, completed the guidance in early 2010. The text was published in the June 2010 issue of *World Psychiatry*, the official journal of the WPA [1], and was posted on the Association's Web site. The guidance has since been translated into several languages, and all the translations have been uploaded on to the same Web site. The document is being extremely well received by the WPA Member Societies (i.e. national psychiatric societies) and by the psychiatric community, and there are already indications that it is being perused by administrators and policy makers from several countries.

Although the steps, obstacles, and mistakes to avoid in the implementation of community mental health care are very similar worldwide, there are regional and national differences, depending on a variety of factors, including the availability of human and financial resources, the level of priority assigned to mental health care by local administrators, and the attitudes of the general population towards mental disorders. It was therefore felt necessary to complement the WPA guidance with documents that delineate the mental health scenario in the various regions of the world and to provide specific recommendations for the development of community mental health services in those regions. A series of papers focusing on the implementation of community mental health care in Africa, Australasia and South Pacific, Europe, North America, Latin America and Caribbean, South Asia, and East and South-East Asia was therefore commissioned and is being published in *World Psychiatry*.

The present volume represents an extension of that series, providing an overview of mental health policies, plans, and programs, a summary of relevant research efforts, a critical appraisal of community mental health service components, and a discussion of the key challenges, obstacles, and lessons learned in the various regions of the world, followed by some recommendations for the future, based on evidence and experience.

We believe that this book represents a very useful resource for all mental health professionals and for all policy makers involved in the mental health field. They will find here not only a picture of the current situation (which can be found, although in bits and pieces, elsewhere) and an outline of the principles of community mental health care (also available in many international documents), but also (and this is unique) a distillate of the experience of several professionals who have been active in community mental health care for decades and are willing to share what they have learned with their colleagues worldwide. The book is recommended to residents in psychiatry and trainees in other mental health professions, who will find it a treasure trove of information and ideas not generally available in textbooks or manuals used in their training.

Professor Mario Maj
President of the World Psychiatric Association

Reference

[1] Thornicroft G, Alem A, Dos Santos RA, et al. WPA guidance on steps, obstacles and mistakes to avoid in the implementation of community mental health care. World Psychiatry 2010;9:67–77.

Acknowledgements

The work which led to this book was commissioned by Professor Mario Maj, President of the World Psychiatric Association, and we are most grateful to Professor Maj for his strong support in establishing the Task Force which undertook it. The authors are pleased to acknowledge the rich contributions of all members of the regional teams that contributed to the various chapters, as given in the List of Contributors.

SECTION 1
Introduction

CHAPTER 1

Global mental health: the context

Introduction

Mental health problems are common, with over 25% of people worldwide developing one or more mental disorders at some point in their life [1]. They make an important contribution to the global burden of disease, as measured by disability-adjusted life years (DALYs). In 2004, for example, neuropsychiatric disorders accounted for 13.1% of all DALYs worldwide, with unipolar depressive disorder alone contributing 4.3% towards total DALYs. In addition, 2.1% of total deaths worldwide were directly attributed to neuropsychiatric disorders. Suicide contributed a further 1.4% towards total deaths, with 86% of all suicides being committed in low- and middle-income countries (LAMICs) each year [2]. A systematic review of psychological autopsy studies of suicide reported a median prevalence of mental disorder in suicide completers of 91% [3]. Life expectancy is up to 20 years lower in people with mental health problems than in those without, due to their higher levels of physical illnesses and far poorer health care [4]. Mental health problems therefore place a substantial burden on individuals and their families worldwide, in terms of both diminished quality of life and reduced life expectancy. The provision of any (let alone high-quality) mental health care is vital in reducing this burden [5].

It is in this context that the aim of this book is to present guidance on the steps, obstacles and mistakes to be avoided in the implementation of community mental health care, and to make realistic and achievable recommendations for the development and implementation of community-oriented mental health care worldwide over the next 10 years. We intend that this guidance will be of practical use to the whole range of mental health and public health practitioners at all levels, including policy makers, commissioners, funders, nongovernmental organizations (NGOs), service users and carers. Although a global approach has been taken, the focus

Community Mental Health: putting policy into practice globally, First Edition. Graham Thornicroft, Maya Semrau, Atalay Alem, Robert E. Drake, Hiroto Ito, Jair Mari, Peter McGeorge, and R. Thara. © 2011 John Wiley & Sons, Ltd. Published 2011 by John Wiley & Sons, Ltd.

is mainly upon LAMICs, as this is where challenges are most severe and most pronounced.

What is community-oriented mental health care?

How can we understand and define community-oriented mental health care? Historically speaking, in the more economically developed countries, mental health service provision has been divided into three periods [6]:

1 The rise of the asylum (from around 1880 to 1955), which was defined by the construction of large asylums that were far removed from the populations they served.

2 The decline of the asylum or "deinstitutionalization" (after around 1955), characterized by a rise in community-based mental health services that were closer to the populations they served.

3 The reform of mental health services according to an evidence-based approach, balancing and integrating elements of both community and hospital services [6–8].

One particular approach that can be useful is the "Balanced Care Model". This is the view that there is no strong evidence that a comprehensive mental health service can be provided with inpatient services alone, nor with community services alone. Rather there needs to be a careful balance of community-based and hospital-based care. The precise mixture of these elements needed will be quite specific to any particular time and place. Nevertheless, the Balanced Care Model is based upon a set of fundamental principles, namely that services should:

• be close to home
• provide interventions for disabilities *and* for symptoms
• be specific to the individual needs
• reflect the priorities of service users
• include both mobile and static services.

In practice these principles will usually mean that most mental health and related services will need to be provided in settings close to the populations served, with hospital stays being reduced as far as possible (in number and duration), and that over time a progressively greater proportion of the mental health budget is spent upon community rather than hospital services [9].

The resources available in LAMICs are so far below those in high-income countries that the Balanced Care Model is organized in a tiered way to indicate service developments that are feasible and realistic at difference levels of resource. For example, the number of psychiatrists per 100 000 population is 5.5–20.0 in Europe and 0.05 in Africa, while there are 87 beds for the same population in Europe compared with 0.34 in Africa, and the proportion of the total health budget dedicated to mental health is 5–12% in Europe and less than 1% on average in Africa. Therefore, to take each resource level in turn:

1 In low-resource settings, the focus is on establishing and improving the capacity of primary health care facilities to deliver mental health care, with limited specialist back-up. Most mental health assessment and treatment occurs, if at all, in primary health care settings or in relation to traditional/religious healers. For example, in Ethiopia, most care is provided within the family or close community of neighbors and relatives: only 33% of people with persistent major depressive disorder reach either primary health care or traditional healers [10, 11].

2 In medium-resource settings, in addition to primary care mental health services, an extra layer of general adult mental health services can be developed. This consists of all of the following five categories: outpatient/ambulatory clinics; community mental health teams; acute inpatient services; community-based residential care; and work, occupation and rehabilitation services (see Appendix A for further descriptions of these services).

3 In high-resource countries, in addition to the services indicated for points 1 and 2, as more resources become available, more specialized services can be provided, in the same five categories. These may include, for instance, specialized outpatient and ambulatory clinics, assertive community treatment teams, intensive case management, early intervention teams, crisis resolution teams, crisis housing, community residential care, acute day hospitals, day hospitals, nonmedical day centers, and recovery/employment/rehabilitation services. It is this Balanced Care Model that is used here as the overall framework in considering community-oriented care. This model is described in more detail in Chapter 10.

In low-resource settings, community-oriented care will be characterized by:

- A focus on population and public health needs.
- Case finding and detection in the community.
- Locally accessible services (i.e. accessible in less than half a day).
- Community participation and decision-making in the planning and provision of mental health care systems.
- Self-help and service-user empowerment for individuals and families.
- Mutual assistance and/or peer support of service users.
- Initial treatment by primary care and/or community staff.
- Stepped care options for referral to specialist staff and/or hospital beds if necessary.
- Back-up supervision and support from specialist mental health services.
- Interfaces with NGOs (for instance in relation to rehabilitation).

- Networks at each level, including between different services, the community, and traditional and/or religious healers.

Community-oriented care, therefore, draws on a wide range of practitioners, providers, care and support systems (both professional and nonprofessional), though particular components may play a greater or lesser role in different settings depending on the local context and the available resources, particularly trained staff.

Fundamental values and human rights

Underpinning the successful implementation of community-oriented mental health care is a set of principles that relate on the one hand to the value of community and on the other to the importance of self-determination and the rights of people with mental illness as persons and citizens [12, 13]. Community mental health services emphasize the importance of treating and enabling people to live in the community in a way that maintains their connection with their families, friends, work, and community. In this process it acknowledges and supports the person's goals and strengths to further his/her recovery in his/her own community [14].

A fundamental principle supporting these values is the notion of people having equitable access to services in their own locality in the "least restrictive environment". While recognizing the fact that some people are significantly impaired by their illness, a community mental health service seeks to foster the service user's self-determination and his/her participation in processes involving decisions related to his/her treatment. Given the importance of families in providing support and key relationships, their participation (with the permission of the service user) in the processes of assessment, treatment planning, and follow-up is also a key value in a community model of service delivery.

Various conventions identify and aim to protect the rights of service users as persons and citizens, including the recently ratified United Nations (UN) Convention on the Rights of Persons with Disability (UNCRPD) [15] and more specific charters such as the UN Principles for the Protection of Persons with Mental Illness and for the Improvement of Mental Care, adopted in 1991 [16].

These and other international, regional, and national documents specify the right of the person to be treated without discrimination and on the same basis as other persons; the presumption of legal capacity unless incapacity can be clearly proven; and the need to involve persons with disabilities in policy and service development, and in decision-making which directly affects them [16]. This book has been written to explicitly align with the requirements of the UNCRPD and associated treaties and conventions.

How information has been gathered for this book

This book has been produced by taking into account the key ethical principles, the relevant evidence, and the combined experience of the authors and their many collaborators. For the Africa region, for example, an expert survey was conducted to collect information on the experience of colleagues who have been active in the last decade in developing mental health services. In relation to the available scientific evidence, systematic literature searches were undertaken to identify peer-reviewed and grey literature concerning the structure, functioning, and effectiveness of community mental health services or obstacles to their implementation. These literature searches were organized for the World Health Organization's (WHO) regions, reflecting the locations of the book's authors. Yet there are limitations to this approach; in particular, the WHO Eastern Mediterranean region was not fully represented. Also, as this book focuses upon adult mental health services, it does not directly address the service needs of people with dementia or intellectual impairment, or of children with mental disorders.

Systematic literature searches

Systematic literature searches were conducted for the different WHO regions to identify peer-reviewed and grey literature. It was important to search for grey literature for two reasons. First, an underrepresentation in databases of indexed journals of publications from LAMICs has been identified [17, 18]; work conducted in such countries may therefore be found elsewhere. Second, reports produced by government bodies and charities concerning the development of community mental health services may contain valuable information concerning lessons learned, but are unlikely to be found in databases of peer-reviewed journals.

A search strategy was devised with the help of a specialist mental health librarian. This was carried out in each WHO region according to local expertise and resources. For each region, searches were limited to studies in humans, studies conducted in the relevant countries, and studies published in languages spoken by the relevant authors; for instance, for the chapter on the European region, studies were limited to those published in English, and for the African region studies in English and French were included.

Table 1.1 provides an overview of the search methods for each region. As an example of the regional searches, a detailed overview of the search methodology employed in the Africa region is provided in Box 1.1.

Table 1.1 Sources searched by regional authors to identify peer-reviewed and grey literature concerning the structure, functioning, and effectiveness, or obstacles to implementation, of community mental health services.

WHO region	Database searched	Other electronic searches	Supplementary searches	Other
Africa	MEDLINE, EMBASE, PsycINFO	Google	Reference lists of included articles Hand searches of the last five years of: *African Journal of Psychiatry*, *South African Journal of Psychiatry*, *International Psychiatry*	Questionnaire survey of regional experts. 21 responses (n) from: Cote D'Ivoire (1), Kenya (3), Liberia (1), Malawi (1), Niger (1), Nigeria (3), South Africa (3), Sudan (1), Tanzania (1), Uganda (3), Zimbabwe (2), NGO (1)
Australasia and South Pacific	MEDLINE	Google	Reference lists of included articles	
East and South East Asia	MEDLINE	Google	Reference lists of included articles	Email survey of regional experts in China, Indonesia, Japan, Singapore, South Korea, and Thailand
Europe	MEDLINE, EMBASE, PsycINFO	Google, OpenSIGLE, Web of Knowledge (ISI), WorldCat Dissertations and Theses (OCLC)	Reference lists of included articles	
Latin America	MEDLINE, Lilacs, EMBASE and SciELO	WHO, PAHO, Google, Mental Health Associations, World Psychiatry Association, Ministry of Health of LAC countries	Reference lists of included articles	
North America	MEDLINE, PsycINFO	WHO, World Psychiatry	Corrigan et al. 2008 [19]	
South Asia	MEDLINE		Reference lists of included articles	

Key texts, such as WHO reports [32–34], papers published by the current authors [6, 7, 22], and a special issue of the *Lancet* in 2007 concerning global mental health [26–31], were also sourced by all regional authors. (NGO, Nongovernmental organization; PAHO, Pan American Health Organization; LAC, Latin American and Caribbean.)

Box 1.1   Literature search strategy for the Africa region.

MEDLINE, EMBASE and PsycINFO databases were searched using the following search terms: (community mental health/or community mental health centers/or community mental health services/) OR (community care.mp. [mp = title, abstract, heading word, table of contents, key concepts]) OR (mental health care provision.mp. [mp = title, abstract, heading word, table of contents, key concepts]). The following key words were also used to search for relevant articles: (community mental health teams OR CHMT OR case management OR assertive community treatment OR assertive community outreach OR early intervention OR home treat* OR crisis hous* OR crisis resolution OR crisis support OR acute care OR acute day care OR inpatient unit* OR resident* OR balanced care OR primary care/(Subject heading) OR rehabilitation OR outpatient OR ambulatory) AND (mental OR psychiatr*) AND (africa or african).lo.(In MEDLINE and EMBASE, the suffix "cp" (country of publication) rather than "lo" (location) was used). The search was limited to English or French publications. Publications relating to services for children, the elderly, substance misuse, or people with intellectual disability were excluded. We also excluded mental health service interventions in a post-conflict context. Obtained abstracts were independently assessed for relevance by two contributors. We then attempted to obtain the full papers for all abstracts designated "relevant" or "possibly relevant" by either reviewer.

Google was searched on 02/11/2009 using an advanced search as follows:

Words: community mental health (in the text of the page) AND individual African countries. Limits: PDFs (hits in any language, but only selected English or French pages). Searched for papers relating to "development" or "evaluation" of overall mental health services (i.e. not specific interventions or groups). NOT children/adolescents. Newsletters and journalistic pieces excluded. If >300 hits, then searched within hits for "development".

In addition, references of obtained articles were checked for other relevant articles. The last five years of the following journals were manually checked for relevant articles: *African Journal of Psychiatry*, *South African Journal of Psychiatry* and *International Psychiatry*.

MEDLINE was searched for every region. Other databases searched were EMBASE, PsycINFO, LILACS, SciELO, Web of Knowledge (ISI), World-Cat Dissertations and Theses (OCLC), and OpenSigle. Searches, adapted for each database, were for MESH terms and text words relating to community mental health services and severe mental illness. Other electronic, nonindexed sources, such as the WHO, Pan American Health Organization (PAHO), WPA, other mental health associations, and country-specific Ministry of Health Web sites were also searched. Google was searched for PDFs published in European and African countries which contained the words "community mental health". The titles, abstracts, or Web pages of identified grey literature were scanned in order to identify publications relating to the development of community mental health services.

Electronic searches were supplemented by searches of the reference lists of all selected articles. Hand searches of issues from the past five years of three key journals relevant to Africa (*African Journal of Psychiatry, South African Journal of Psychiatry,* and *International Psychiatry*) were also conducted. In addition, key texts were identified: these included relevant papers and book chapters published by authors of the current work [20–25] and a special edition of the *Lancet* on Global Mental Health [26–31]. WHO publications which provide information regarding community mental health services worldwide were also sourced [5, 32–34].

Expert survey

For the Africa region, original research was conducted in order to supplement published data. Twenty-one regional experts completed a semi-structured, self-report questionnaire concerning their experience in implementing community mental health care in sub-Saharan Africa. The experts were from eleven countries and one NGO active in several countries across sub-Saharan Africa. Further details of the questionnaire are given in Box 1.2 (see also Appendix B for survey questions).

Box 1.2   Regional expert questionnaire in the Africa region.

The main aim of the questionnaire was to obtain details of experience implementing community mental health care in sub-Saharan Africa, in order to supplement information available from published reports. We made use of the World Psychiatric Association regional Africa meeting, held in Abuja in October 2009, as a starting point to contact leaders in mental health care from across sub-Saharan Africa. The snowballing technique was employed by asking respondents to recommend further contacts. Additionally, we contacted the WHO Regional Office for Africa in Brazzaville, Congo, to ask for details of any innovative programs of mental health care being implemented in the region.

The questionnaire is detailed in Appendix B. A French translation was sent to contacts in French-speaking countries.

We attempted to contact 41 experts and received 21 responses to our questionnaire, from the following countries: Cote D'Ivoire (1), Kenya (3), Liberia (1), Malawi (1), Niger (1), Nigeria (3), South Africa (3), Sudan (1), Tanzania (1), Uganda (3), Zimbabwe (2) and an NGO active in several countries across sub-Saharan Africa. We were unsuccessful in obtaining any response from a further six countries in sub-Saharan Africa. We made use of our own knowledge of the situation in Ethiopia, supported by discussions with Ministry of Health officials. A limitation of the study is that we did not have contacts in every African country.

Of the respondents, nine were from academic departments (seven of whom were Professors or Heads of Department), three were involved in national mental health programs, one worked with the WHO and another as mental health advisor to the Ministry of Health, three were national or regional representatives of mental health organizations, and two respondents were from mental health NGOs.

Key points in this chapter

- Mental health problems are common and pose a huge burden for populations, patients, and their families worldwide.
- This book uses the Balanced Care Model in considering community-oriented care, in which services are provided in community settings close to the populations served, and hospital stays are reduced as far as possible.
- Underpinning community-based mental health care are the principles of human rights and equitable access to services for patients in their own locality in as least restrictive an environment as possible, in particular the new overarching human rights of the United Nations: the Convention on the Rights of Persons with Disabilities.
- Information was gathered for this book from literature reviews for different WHO global regions, from the combined experience of the authors and their collaborators, from an expert survey in the Africa region, and in base upon key conventions relating to human rights.

References

[1] World Health Organization. The World Health Report 2001—Mental Health: New Understanding, New Hope. 2001.

[2] World Health Organization. The Global Burden of Disease: 2004 Update. 2008.

[3] Cavanagh JT, Carson AJ, Sharpe M, Lawrie SM. Psychological autopsy studies of suicide: a systematic review. Psychological Medicine 2003;33:395–405.

[4] Chwastiak LA, Tek C. The Unchanging Mortality Gap for People with Schizophrenia. Lancet 2009;374(9690):590–2.

[5] World Health Organization. Mental Health Gap Action Programme: Scaling Up Care for Mental, Neurological, and Substance Use Disorders. 2008.

[6] Thornicroft G, Tansella M. What are the arguments for community-based mental health care? Copenhagen: WHO Regional Office for Europe; 2003.

[7] Thornicroft G, Tansella M. Components of a modern mental health service: A pragmatic balance of community and hospital care—Overview of systematic evidence. British Journal of Psychiatry 2004;185:283–90.

[8] Thornicroft G, Tansella M. Better Mental Health Care. Cambridge: Cambridge University Press; 2009.

[9] Thornicroft G, Tansella M. Balancing community-based and hospital-based mental health care. World Psychiatry 2002;1:84–90.

[10] Hanlon C, Medhin G, Alem A, Araya M, Abdulahi A, Tesfaye M, et al. Measuring common mental disorders in women in Ethiopia: Reliability and construct validity of the Comprehensive Psychopathological Rating Scale. Social Psychiatry and Psychiatric Epidemiology 2008;43:653–9.

[11] Fekadu A, O'Donovan MC, Alem A, Kepede D, Church S, Johns L, et al. Validity of the concept of minor depression in a developing country setting. Journal of Nervous and Mental Disease 2008;196:22–8.

[12] Bartlett P, Lewis O, Thorold O. Mental disability and the European Convention on Human Rights. Leiden: Martinus Nijhoff; 2006.

[13] Thornicroft G, Tansella M. Translating ethical principles into outcome measures for mental health service research. Psychological Medicine 1999;29:761–7.

[14] Slade M. Personal recovery and mental illness: A guide for mental health professionals. Cambridge: Cambridge University Press; 2009.

[15] United Nations. Convention on the rights of persons with disabilities. New York: United Nations; 2006.

[16] United Nations. UN principles for the protection of persons with mental illness and for the improvement of mental health care. New York: United Nations; 1992.

[17] Kieling C, Herman H, Patel V, Mari JD. Indexation of psychiatric journals from low and middle-income countries: a survey and a case study. World Psychiatry 2009;8(1):40–4.

[18] Mari J, Patel V, Kieling C, Razzouk D, Tyrer P, Herman H. The 5/95 gap in the indexation of psychiatric journals of low- and middle-income countries. Acta Psychiatrica Scandinavica 2010;121(2):152–6.

[19] Corrigan PW, Mueser KT, Bond GR, Drake RE, Solomon P. The Principles and Practice of Psychiatric Rehabilitation. New York: Guilford Press; 2008.

[20] Mbuba CK, Newton CR. Packages of care for epilepsy in low- and middle-income countries. PLoS Medicine 2009;6(10):e1000162.

[21] Patel V, Simon G, Chowdary N, Kaaya S, Araya R. Packages of care for depression in low- and middle-income countries. PLoS Medicine 2009;6(10):e1000159.

[22] Thornicroft G, Tansella M, Law A. Steps, challenges and lessons in developing community mental health care. World Psychiatry 2008;7:87–92.

[23] Patel V, Thornicroft G. Packages of care for mental, neurological, and substance use disorders in low- and middle-income countries. PLoS Medicine 2009;6: e1000160.

[24] Benegal V, Chand PK, Obot IS. Packages of care for alcohol use disorders in low- and middle-income countries. PLoS Medicine 2009;6(10):e1000170.

[25] de Jesus Mari J, Razzouk D, Thara R, Eaton J, Thornicroft G. Packages of care for schizophrenia in low- and middle-income countries. PLoS Medicine 2009;6(10):e1000165.

[26] Prince M, Patel V, Saxena S, Maj M, Maselko J, Phillips MR, et al. No health without mental health. Lancet 2007 Sep 8;370(9590):859–77.

[27] Patel V, Araya R, Chatterjee S, Chisholm D, Cohen A, De SM, et al. Treatment and prevention of mental disorders in low-income and middle-income countries. Lancet 2007 Sep 15;370(9591):991–1005.

[28] Saxena S, Thornicroft G, Knapp M, Whiteford H. Resources for mental health: scarcity, inequity, and inefficiency. Lancet 2007 Sep 8;370(9590): 878–89.

[29] Jacob KS, Sharan P, Mirza I, Garrido-Cumbrera M, Seedat S, Mari JJ, et al. Mental health systems in countries: where are we now? Lancet 2007 Sep 22;370(9592):1061–77.

[30] Saraceno B, Van OM, Batniji R, Cohen A, Gureje O, Mahoney J, et al. Barriers to improvement of mental health services in low-income and middle-income countries. Lancet 2007 Sep 29;370(9593):1164–74.

[31] Chisholm D, Flisher AJ, Lund C, Patel V, Saxena S, Thornicroft G, et al. Scale up services for mental disorders: a call for action. Lancet 2007 Oct 6;370(9594): 1241–52.

[32] World Health Organization. Mental Health Atlas, revised edition. Geneva: WHO; 2005.

[33] World Health Organization. Mental Health Systems in Selected Low- and Middle-Income Countries: A WHO-AIMS Cross-National Analysis. Geneva: WHO; 2009.

[34] World Health Organization. Policies and Practices for Mental Health in Europe—Meeting the Challenges. Geneva: WHO; 2008.

CHAPTER 2
Description of the world regions

Introduction

This chapter provides an overview of the WHO regions covered in this book: Africa, Australasia and South Pacific, Europe, Latin America and Caribbean, South Asia, and East and South-East Asia. These regions, shown in Figure 2.1, are discussed in turn. Although the book also covers North America (which includes the United Stated of America and Canada), this region is not discussed in this or the next chapter.

Africa

The Africa region of the WHO includes 46 countries (i.e. all countries on the African continent, apart from Morocco, Tunisia, Libya, Egypt, Sudan, and Somalia), classified into the following World Bank income categories: low-income (n = 30), lower middle-income (n = 8), upper middle-income (n = 5) and high-income (n = 1). The total population of Africa was estimated to be approximately 818 million people in 2008, with an average growth rate of 2.5% per annum [1].

The burden of communicable diseases remains high in most African countries, for example with an average HIV prevalence of 5.0% across the continent and life expectancy at birth of only 51.5 years [1]. Mental health therefore vies for its place amongst other compelling and competing public health priorities, especially in relation to the Millennium Development Goals [2]. However, funding for mental health care in the African region is disproportionately low when compared to the associated burden of mental disorder [3]. Further challenges to the development of mental health services in the Africa region come from the impact of conflicts, natural disasters, and the brain drain of mental health professionals from government services [4].

Community Mental Health: putting policy into practice globally, First Edition. Graham Thornicroft, Maya Semrau, Atalay Alem, Robert E. Drake, Hiroto Ito, Jair Mari, Peter McGeorge, and R. Thara. © 2011 John Wiley & Sons, Ltd. Published 2011 by John Wiley & Sons, Ltd.

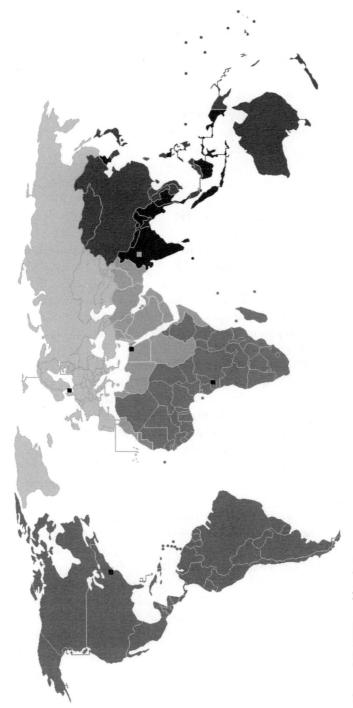

Figure 2.1 WHO world regions.

Table 2.1 Pacific Nations supported by the PIMHnet WHO Pacific Initiative (see Chapters 4 and 5 for details on the PIMHnet WHO Pacific Initiative).

Micronesia	Melanesia	Polynesia
Fed. States of Micronesia	Fiji	Cook Islands
Guam	Papua New Guinea	Niue
Kiribati	Solomon Islands	Samoa (Western)
Nauru	Vanuatu	Tokelau
Northern Marianas		Tonga
Palau		Tuvalu
Wallis and Futuna		New Caledonia
Rep. of Marshall Islands		

Australasia and South Pacific

Together, Australia, New Zealand and the Pacific Nations are commonly referred to as Oceania. The countries of Australia and New Zealand form Australasia. Whilst there are areas within both countries that are impoverished, overall they are classified as high-income countries.

Australia comprises six states and two territories (Northern Territory and Australian Capital Territory), which are collectively referred to as jurisdictions. The population of Australia as of June 2009 was 21 874 000. The indigenous population of Aborigines and Torres Strait Islanders was 517 000 (2.5% of the total). The GDP in 2009 was $959 802 billion AUD (equivalent to 962 111 billion USD).[1] Spending on mental health care in 2008 was $5.32 billion AUD (5.33 billion USD) [5], including by the Australian government ($1.92 billion AUD), jurisdictions ($3.22 billion AUD), and private health insurers ($185 million AUD). 7% of the total expenditure is spent on health care.

The population of New Zealand was estimated at 4.27 million in 2009, with an indigenous Maori population of 625 000 (15% of the population). Pacific Islanders make up 7% of the population. The Asian population (using a broad definition) is growing rapidly, also accounting for 7% of the total population. Those of European stock make up most of the rest of the population. The GDP is $166 825 billion NZD (126 555 billion USD), with spending on mental health care in 2006 amounting to $866 600 million NZD (657 410 million USD)[2] [6]. Spending on mental health care represents close to 11% of the total health care spending.

The Pacific Island states are mainly low-income countries comprising a vast array of island nations broadly grouped within Micronesia, Melanesia,

---

[1] Source: World Bank, November 2010.

[2] In 2009 expenditure was 1.1 billion NZD (830 million USD).

and Polynesia [7] (see Table 2.1). Overall, the population is increasing rapidly. Currently it is estimated at 32 million, with Melanesia having the largest population at around 7 million and Polynesia accounting for 1.2 million. The combined GDP is estimated to be in the range of 106 735 billion USD, with the larger-population countries of Fiji and New Guinea accounting for a substantial proportion of the total.

Based on recent epidemiological surveys, lifetime prevalence rate of mental disorders in Australia is 45%, and in New Zealand 46.6% [8], with annual prevalence rates of around 20% in both countries. There are no comparable data available for Pacific Nations.

Europe

The European region of the WHO comprises 53 countries—more than any other of the WHO's regions. These include (see Tables 3.1, 4.2 and 4.3 in Chapters 3 and 4 for a full list of countries):

- The former EU-15 countries: the fifteen countries that have been part of the European Union (EU) since before 2004.
- Twelve countries that joined the EU from 2004 onwards.
- Eleven countries of the Commonwealth of Independent States (CIS) (which covers most of the former Soviet Union's member states).
- Eight countries from South-Eastern Europe (which includes five member states of the former Yugoslavia, as well as Albania, Georgia, and Turkey).
- Seven additional countries (Andorra, Iceland, Israel, Monaco, Norway, San Marino, and Switzerland).

Countries within the European region are hugely diverse culturally, with a multitude of languages being spoken in the region. Thirty—more than half—of the European countries have been classed as high-income countries by the World Bank [1]. This includes all of the former EU-15 countries, as well as seven of the twelve countries that joined the EU in 2004 or afterwards, one country in South-Eastern Europe (Croatia), and all seven of the remaining (non-classed) countries. The only three low-income countries in the region (Kyrgyzstan, Tajikistan, and Uzbekistan) are members of the CIS, with none of the CIS countries having been classed as high-income. Middle-income countries are spread across the remaining post-2004 EU countries (all of which are upper middle-income), the CIS countries (five of which are lower middle-income), and countries in South-Eastern Europe (most of which are upper middle-income) [1]. Generally speaking, there is therefore an economic divide across Europe, with most of the high-income countries amongst EU countries (in particular the former EU-15 countries) and other primarily

Western countries, and all of the low-income and lower middle-income countries in the non-EU Eastern parts of the region.

Mental health problems are common across Europe: each year over 25% of people in the region are estimated to experience a mental disorder, and around 6% may require mental health care [9]. Mental health problems therefore have a huge economic and social impact in Europe, with neuropsychiatric disorders accounting for 19.1% of all disability-adjusted life-years (DALYs) in the region in 2004, and 39% of all first-ranked cause of years lived with disability (YLD) [10]. Unipolar depression alone is the third leading cause of DALYs in Europe (after ischaemic heart disease and cerebrovascular disease), accounting for 5.6% of DALYs in the region in 2004 [10]. At a prevalence rate of 14.01 per 100 000 population across the region in 2007 [11], and contributing 2% of total DALYs and 1.6% of all deaths in 2004 [10], suicide rates are also high across the European region. In the former EU-15 countries, around 3–4 % of the gross national product has been estimated to be ultimately due to mental health problems (Gabriel and Liimatainen, 2000, in [12]).

Latin America and Caribbean

The WHO region of the Americas includes 34 Latin American and Caribbean (LAC) countries, covering an area of 21 000 000 km^2: Mexico in North America, seven countries in Central America, thirteen countries in South America, and thirteen Caribbean countries. The region is characterized by great cultural and economic diversity. Although Spanish is the main language spoken in sixteen countries, other languages are also spoken widely, including English in eight countries, and Portuguese, French, and Dutch in three countries each. The total population is approximately 600 million, mostly resident in urban areas, and predominately Roman Catholic. However, there is a vast ethnic diversity, mainly compounded by Amerindians, Mestizos, blacks and whites.

Over the past decade, most LAC countries have experienced economic and scientific growth [13, 14], a political shift from dictatorial to democratic regimes, civil-rights movements, and the implementation of national health policies, leading to an increase in life expectancy and a reduction in infant mortality [15]. Although 44% of countries are middle-income countries and 35% are upper middle-income countries, economic inequality is markedly high, as expressed by the GINI coefficient (measuring inequalities in wealth distribution; the median figure of countries is 0.55), similar to many low-income African countries. Approximately one-third of people live below the poverty line in LAC countries [16].

Colombia, Brazil, and Mexico have the greatest number of cities, with high rates of inequality and GINI coefficients over 0.6, much higher than the international warning line (0.4). LAC countries share some common problems, such as the high level of violence, drug trafficking, high levels of alcohol consumption, and high rates of illiteracy and unemployment. Local conflict, wars, and natural disasters are predominant in countries of Central America and the Caribbean. Prevalence of mental disorders is high in the region: one-year prevalence varies from 20 to 25%, with a predominance of generalized anxiety disorder (3.4%), alcohol dependence (5.7%), and depression (4.9%) [17].

South Asia

The WHO South Asia region includes the southern region of the Asian continent. For the purposes of this book, the sub-Himalayan countries of Bangladesh, Bhutan, India, the Maldives, Nepal, Pakistan, and Sri Lanka have been included in the region, as well as Afghanistan.

South Asia is home to 23% of the world's population, making it the most populous and most densely populated geographical region in the world. Many (40%) of the poorest people in the world live here, and its relatively young population is one of the least literate and most malnourished in the world. The region has often seen conflicts and political instability, including wars between the region's two nuclear-armed states, Pakistan and India.

One-fifth of all patients with psychiatric disorders worldwide live in the South Asia region. Despite vast cultural, religious, geographical, and political diversities, factors influencing mental health are similar throughout the region. Prevalence and diagnoses of mental disorders are roughly the same across South Asian countries, with a total prevalence of around 10–12%. The total number of mentally ill people in the region is around 150–200 million.

The characteristic feature of South Asian countries is the diversity in ethnicity, language, religion, economy, and politics. More than 2000 ethnic communities and populations are present, ranging in population size from hundreds of millions to small tribal groups, speaking many different languages. With almost 422 million people using it, Hindi is the most widely spoken language in the region, followed by Bengali with about 210 million speakers [18]. Urdu is another major language spoken in the subcontinent, especially in Pakistan and India. English also dominates South Asia, especially within advanced education and government administration. Hinduism and Islam, and in some countries Buddhism, are the dominant religions. Other Indian religions and Christianity are also practiced by a significant number of people.

Sri Lanka has the highest GDP per capita in the region [19], whilst Nepal and Afghanistan have the lowest. India is the largest economy in the

Table 2.2 Countries in East and South-East Asia covered in this book.

	Population[a]	Languages	GDP[b]	Health expenditure[c]	Health care system
Brunei	0.4	Malay	12.3	1.9	Public/private sector
Cambodia	13.4	Khmer	8.7	5.9	Public sector
China, including Hong Kong	1321.1	Chinese	3382.4	4.6	Public sector
Indonesia	224.9	Indonesian	432.1	2.5	Public/private sector
Japan	127.8	Japanese	4384.4	8.1	More private hospitals (80%) Public health centres
Laos	6.1	Lao	4.1	4.0	Public/private sector
Malaysia	26.8	Malay, Chinese, Tamil, and English	186.7	4.3	Public/private sector
Mongolia	2.6	Mongolian	3.9	5.7	Public/private sector
Myanmar	57.6	Myanmar	19.6	2.2	Public/private sector
Philippines	88.6	Filipino, English	144.1	3.8	Public/private sector
Singapore	4.6	Malay, English, Chinese, and Tamil	167.0	3.3	Private/public sectors Public community care
South Korea	48.5	Korean	1049.3	6.4	More private hospitals
Thailand	65.7	Thai	246.1	3.5	Public/private sector
Timor-Leste	1.0	Tetung and Portuguese	0.4	17.7	
Viet Nam	85.2	Vietnamese	71.1	6.6	Public sector

Data from the World Bank Group.
[a]in millions, from International Monetary Fund, World Economic Outlook Database [26].
[b]in billion US dollars, from International Monetary Fund, World Economic Outlook Database [26].
[c]% of GDP, from the World Bank Group.

region [20], followed by Pakistan (which has the third highest GDP per capita in the region [21]), and then Bangladesh. According to the World Bank, 70% of the South Asian population and about 75% of South Asia's poor live in rural areas and mostly rely on agriculture for their livelihood [22]. The rapid increase in food grain productivity in the 1970s and 1980s made possible by the "Green Revolution" improved food security and increased rural wages. As a consequence, the rural poverty rate has declined significantly. In India, for example, it fell from about 53% in

1977/78 to 26% in 1999/2000. However, according to the Global Hunger Index, South Asia still has one of the highest child malnutrition rates in the world [23], with the number of child deaths in 2008 being around 2.1 million [21]. High illiteracy rates in villages have been highlighted as another major issue needing more government attention.

East and South-East Asia

East and South-East Asia covers a wide area, with fifteen countries (four in East Asia and eleven in South-East Asia) included in the region for the purposes of this book (see Table 2.2). It is a heterogeneous region with marked cultural, religious, and socioeconomic diversity. In terms of GDP, the total health expenditure of countries within the region ranges from 1.9 to 17.7% (see Table 2.2). Throughout the region, in both low-income and high-income settings, countries devote only a small fraction of their total health budgets to mental health (less than 1% and 5%, respectively [24]). Increasing qualitative and quantitative health care demands are placing pressures on governments in countries where public-sector health care once dominated private care [25]. Because of varied historical backgrounds and colonial heritages, health care systems diverge even among neighboring countries.

Key points in this chapter

- Seven regions are covered in this book: Africa, Australasia and South Pacific, Europe, North America, Latin America and Caribbean, South Asia, and East and South-East Asia.
- There are huge cultural and economic differences both within and across regions.
- What unites the countries within these regions is that, compared with the global burden of disease attribute to neuropsychiatric disorders, a very low proportion of the total health budget is spent on mental health care.

References

[1] The World Bank. Country Classification. http://www.worldbank.org/ 2009 July (cited 9 A.D. Dec 30).

[2] Prince M, Patel V, Saxena S, Maj M, Maselko J, Phillips MR, et al. No health without mental health. Lancet 2007;370(9590):859–77.

[3] Saxena S, Thornicroft G, Knapp M, Whiteford H. Resources for mental health: scarcity, inequity, and inefficiency. Lancet 2007;370(9590):878–89.

[4] Saraceno B, van Ommeren M, Batniji R, et al. Barriers to improvement of mental health services in low-income and middle-income countries. Lancet 2007; 370(9593):1164–74.

[5] Department of Health and Aging. National Mental Health Report. Canberra: Commonwealth of Australia; 2010.

[6] Mental Health Commission (MHC). Report on Progress 2004/2005. Wellington, New Zealand; 2006.

[7] Hughes F. Report to the World Health Organisation on Developing a Technical Support Programme for the Organisation of Mental Health Services in the Western Pacific Region. Mary Finlayson, editor. 2005. Auckland, New Zealand, Centre for Mental Health Research, Policy and Service Development. Patrick Firkin.

[8] Oakley-Browne MA, Wells JE, Scott KM. Te Rau Hinengaro: The New Zealand Mental Health Survey. Mental Health, editor. Wellington; 2006. Ministry of Health.

[9] Wahlbeck K, Huber M. European Centre Policy Brief April 2009: Access to Health Care for People with Mental Disorders in Europe. 2009.

[10] World Health Organization. The Global Burden of Disease: 2004 Update. 2008.

[11] World Health Organization. European Health for All Database. Geneva: WHO; 2009.

[12] Knapp M, McDaid D, Mossialos E, Thornicroft G. Mental Health Policy and Practice Across Europe: An Overview. In: Knapp M, McDaid D, Mossialos E, Thornicroft G, editors. Mental Health Policy and Practice Across Europe. Maidenhead: Open University Press; 2007. pp. 1–14.

[13] Razzouk D, Gallo C, Olifson S, Zorzetto R, Fiestas F, Poletti G, et al. Challenges to reduce the '10/90 gap': mental health research in Latin American and Caribbean countries. Acta Psychiatrica Scandinavica 2008;118:490–8.

[14] Razzouk D, Zorzetto R, Dubugras MT, Gerolin J, Mari Jde J. Leading countries in mental health research in Latin America and the Caribbean. Revista Brasileira de Psiquiatria 2007;29:118–22.

[15] Alarcon RD, Aguilar-Gaxiola SA. Mental health policy developments in Latin America. Bulletin of the World Health Organization 2000;78(4):483–90.

[16] Alarcon RD. Mental health and mental health care in Latin America. World Psychiatry 2003;2(1):54–6.

[17] Kohn R, Levav I, de Almeida JM, Vicente B, Andrade L, Caraveo-Anduaga JJ, et al. [Mental disorders in Latin America and the Caribbean: a public health priority]. Revista Panamericana de Salud Pública 2005;18:229–40.

[18] Office of the Registrar General and Census Commissioner of India. Census of India. 2001.

[19] The World Bank. Sri Lanka at a Glance. 2010.

[20] The World Bank. India at a Glance. 2010.

[21] The World Bank. Pakistan at a Glance. 2010.

[22] The World Bank. Agriculture in South Asia. 2010.

[23] International Food Policy Research Institute (IFPRI). Global Hunger Index. 2010.

[24] Saxena S, Sharan P, Saraceno B. Budget and financing of mental health services: baseline information on 89 Countries from WHO's Project Atlas. The Journal of Mental Health Policy and Economics 2003;6:135–43.

[25] Ramesh M, Wu X. Realigning public and private health care in Southeast Asia. The Pacific Review 2008;21:171–87.

[26] International Monetary Fund. World Economic Outlook Database. 2009.

CHAPTER 3

Overview of mental health policies worldwide

Introduction

This chapter provides an overview of mental health policies and legislation that apply in selected countries in the WHO regions worldwide. The World Psychiatric Association Task Force that undertook the preparatory work for this book was not able to gather such information for all countries, so we present here rich and revealing data about many, but not all, countries of the world.

Europe

Mental Health Declaration and Action Plan

Europe is one of the regions in which there has been considerable progress over the last decade in the development and reform of mental health policies [1]. A significant milestone was the Mental Health Declaration for Europe [2] and the Mental Health Action Plan for Europe [3], which were agreed and signed by all European health ministers at a meeting in Helsinki in January 2005. By signing the Declaration, ministers acknowledged mental health as a priority area, recognized the need for evidence-based mental health policies, defined a broad scope for these policies, and committed themselves to the development, implementation, and reinforcement of such policies. The Action Plan proposed 12 action areas for the development of comprehensive mental health services, along with milestones for each of these areas to be implemented. The main priorities identified were to: (i) foster awareness of mental wellbeing; (ii) tackle stigma, discrimination, and inequality; (iii) develop comprehensive, integrated mental health systems; (iv) provide a competent, effective workforce; and (v) recognize the experience of services users/carers [4].

Community Mental Health: putting policy into practice globally, First Edition. Graham Thornicroft, Maya Semrau, Atalay Alem, Robert E. Drake, Hiroto Ito, Jair Mari, Peter McGeorge, and R. Thara. © 2011 John Wiley & Sons, Ltd. Published 2011 by John Wiley & Sons, Ltd.

Policies and legislation

As a result, mental health has been high on the list of priorities in many European countries in recent years, with most countries in the region having made substantial progress towards achieving the Action Plan's milestones [5]. Most, 83% of, countries in the region now have a mental health policy in place (see Table 3.1), with the latest figures (in 2005) estimating that around 89% of the population in the region was covered by such policies [6]. Similarly, all countries in the European region, apart from Andorra, now have mental health legislation (see Table 3.1), with around 90% of the population in the region being covered by such legislation in 2005 [6, 7] (as a comparison, around 78% of countries worldwide had mental health legislation in place in 2005, with around 69% of the population worldwide covered by such legislation [6]).

However, there are large variations in the content and application of policies and legislation across countries within Europe. Whilst in many countries policies have been updated in recent years to fit in with changing ideas of mental health service provision—with half of the countries with mental health policies in place having either adopted new policies or updated existing policies since 2005 (see Table 3.1)—others are out of date and in need of early modernization [8, 9]. Similarly, although about 40% of countries with mental health legislation have updated their legislation or adopted new legislation since 2005, around one-sixth of countries still have laws that are over 10 years old (see Table 3.1).

Community mental health services

The Mental Health Declaration for Europe [2] included a commitment by health ministers across Europe to develop community-based mental health services as a replacement for large mental institutions. Consequently, with almost one-quarter of countries in Europe having policies, strategies, or plans for the development of community mental health services in place, this is now the area most directly addressed by policies across the region. Similarly, policies, plans, or strategies for the downgrading of large mental hospitals have been developed in around 60% of European countries (see Table 3.1), with countries that have not yet adopted such policies tending to be those in the eastern or south-eastern parts of Europe.

Integration of mental health into primary health care

The Mental Health Declaration for Europe also committed health ministers to the integration of mental health services into primary health care, and emphasized that the successful implementation of community-based mental health services is dependent on this integration [2]. Policies for the integration of mental health into primary care now exist in over two-thirds of countries across the region (see Table 3.1).

Table 3.1 Overview of mental health policies and legislation in the European region.

	Year of most recently approved or updated mental health legislation	Year of most recent mental health policy	Policies, strategies or plans: development of community mental health services	Policies, strategies or plans: downsizing of large mental hospitals	Policies, strategies or plans: mental health in primary health care
Former EU-15					
Austria	after 2005	after 2005	Yes	Yes	Yes
Belgium	after 2005	after 2005	Yes	Yes	Yes
Denmark	after 2005	after 2005	Yes	Yes	Yes
Finland	after 2005	1999–2004	Yes	No	Yes
France	after 2005	after 2005	Yes	Yes	Yes
Germany	after 2005	after 2005	Yes	Yes	Yes
Greece	1999	1999–2004	Yes	Yes	No
Ireland	after 2005	after 2005	Yes	Yes	Yes
Italy	1978	after 2005	Yes	N/A	Yes
Luxembourg	2000	1999–2004	Yes	Yes	Yes
Netherlands	1999–2004	1999	Yes	Yes	Yes
Portugal	1999–2004	after 2005	Yes	Yes	Yes
Spain	after 2005	after 2005	Yes	Yes	Yes
Sweden	2000	before 1998	Yes	Yes	Yes
United Kingdom	after 2005	after 2005	Yes	Yes	Yes
Other EU					
Bulgaria	after 2005	after 2005	Yes	Yes	Yes
Cyprus	1999–2004	after 2005	Yes	Yes	Yes
Czech Republic	after 2005	1999–2004	Yes	Yes	Yes
Estonia	after 2005	No policy	No	No	No
Hungary	1997	1999–2004	Yes	Yes	Yes
Latvia	after 2005	2004	Yes	No	No
Lithuania	after 2005	after 2005	Yes	Yes	Yes
Malta	1981	1994	Yes	Yes	Yes
Poland	after 2005	after 2005	Yes	Yes	Yes
Romania	2002	after 2005	Yes	No	Yes
Slovakia	after 2005	1999–2004	Yes	Yes	Yes
Slovenia	before 1998	1999–2004	No	No	Yes
South-Eastern					
Albania	1996	2003	Yes	Yes	Yes
Bosnia and Herzegovina	2000	after 2005	Yes	Yes	Yes
Croatia	1999–2004	after 2005	Yes	Yes	Yes
Georgia	after 2005	No policy	No	No	No
Montenegro	after 2005	1999–2004	Yes	No	Yes

(Continued)

Table 3.1 Continued.

	Year of most recently approved or updated mental health legislation	Year of most recent mental health policy	Policies, strategies or plans: development of community mental health services	Policies, strategies or plans: downsizing of large mental hospitals	Policies, strategies or plans: mental health in primary health care
Serbia	Has legislation	after 2005	Yes	Yes	Yes
T.F.Y.R. of Macedonia	after 2005	after 2005	Yes	Yes	Yes
Turkey	1999–2004	after 2005	Yes	Yes	Yes
CIS					
Armenia	2004	1994	N/A	N/A	N/A
Azerbaijan	2001	No policy	No	No	No
Belarus	1999	No policy	N/A	N/A	N/A
Kazakhstan	1997	1997	N/A	N/A	N/A
Kyrgyzstan	1999	2000	N/A	N/A	N/A
R. of Moldova	1998	No policy	Yes	No	Yes
Russian Federation	1999–2004	after 2005	Yes	Yes	Yes
Tajikistan	N/A	No policy	N/A	N/A	N/A
Turkmenistan	1993	1995	N/A	N/A	N/A
Ukraine	2000	1988	N/A	N/A	N/A
Uzbekistan	2000	1999–2004	Yes	Yes	Yes
Other					
Andorra	No legislation	No policy	N/A	N/A	N/A
Iceland	1997	No policy	N/A	N/A	N/A
Israel	2000	after 2005	Yes	Yes	Yes
Monaco	1981	Has policy	N/A	N/A	N/A
Norway	after 2005	after 2005	Yes	Yes	Yes
San Marino	Has legislation	No policy	N/A	N/A	N/A
Switzerland	1981	after 2005	Yes	Yes	Yes

N/A: information not available.

Data taken from World Health Organization's publications [5, 6, 10–13]. Where data were conflicting between publications, the most recent source was used.

Note: some countries in Europe—Spain, for instance—have independent regions [5]. Whilst it is acknowledged that these regions may have separate mental health legislation, policies, and service provision in place, any differences within countries are not described further. Rather, it is indicated where policies or legislation exist in any of the regions of a country.

Latin America and the Caribbean

In the region of Latin America and the Caribbean, the Declaration of Caracas was signed in 1990, which targeted the shift from hospital care to community care based on four core principles: (i) the protection of human rights; (ii) the promotion of social inclusion of people with mental disorders; (iii) a decrease in the burden of mental disorders; and (iv) the provision of cost-effective treatments and services. These objectives were identified in order to improve the quality of life of people with mental disorders, and also to integrate mental health into the primary health care system [14, 15]. Over the last few decades, this new model of mental health care has been variously implemented according to local policies and financial resources [16, 17]. Nonetheless, mental health care has not been regarded as an important priority for most of the countries in the region. At the time of the most recent Mental Health Atlas [6, 15], seven countries (20%) still did not have a mental health policy in place, five (14%) did not have a mental health program in place, and six (18%) had no specific legislation for mental health [18].

Africa

The development of policies and legislation has been much slower in the WHO Africa region [19–22]. At the time of the WHO Mental Health Atlas, only half—23 of the 46—countries in the Africa region had a mental health policy in place, with a further six countries being in the process of developing a policy [6]. Twenty of the countries with a mental health policy also had a mental health program. Nine countries had a mental health program in the absence of a policy [23]. Over half of the countries had mental health legislation, although the majority had not been revised recently [24–28].

South Asia

Many countries in South Asia also lack mental health policies and infrastructure [29–31] (see Table 3.2). Mental health policies are present in only a few countries in the region. Furthermore, of the countries that do have mental health legislation in place, with the exception of India (which introduced a policy in 1982), all were developed during the late 1990s and still lack a comprehensive approach. Mental health legislation plays an important role in implementing effective mental health services, particularly

Table 3.2 Overview of mental health policies, laws, plans, and services in the South Asia region.

Country [source]	Mental health policy	Legislation	Mental health plan	Mental health services in primary care	Community mental health services
Afghanistan [56]	National mental health plan used as mental health policy	Afghanistan's Independent Human Rights Commission	Present	Non-existent	Limited
Bangladesh [57]	Incorporated in policy, strategy and action plan for surveillance and prevention of noncommunicable diseases	Draft version prepared but not enacted	Incorporated in strategy and work plan for community-based activities	Present; regular training of primary care personnel exists	Day care facilities, sheltered workshops, and rehabilitation programs for chronic schizophrenics; NGO involvement active
Bhutan [58]	Formulated as part of the country's five-year plan of development	No separate legislation for mental health; clause in Bhutan penal code safeguards the interests of people with mental illness in the criminal justice system	Comprehensive mental health plan exists	Integrated services present; standard treatment manual for health workers includes common mental disorders; common mental disorders included in general health information systems	Pilot efforts have involved traditional healers and religious leaders in surveys for mental illness; training of community workers has been carried out
India [59, 60]	No mental health policy; national health policy addresses mental health care	Mental health act enacted in 1987; National Human Rights Commission; document on human rights and mental health	National mental health program present; district mental health program	Mental health program aimed at integrating mental health care with primary care	Organized community care initiatives present; NGO involvement active

Maldives [61]	No mental health policy	No legislation	No plan	Mental health is not part of primary health care	Community health worker training has a mental health component; NGO involvement in rehabilitation of disabled children, substance users
Nepal [62]	Present	Draft mental health legislation submitted to ministry of health; no human rights review body	No separate mental health plan	Integration in 7 of 75 districts	One NGO is running a community mental health service in 7 districts
Pakistan [63]	Present	Present	Incorporated in national action plan for noncommunicable diseases	Sparse	Phased development of community mental health program; extensive training of administrators, school teachers, and faith healers
Sri Lanka [64]	Present	In preparation	No plan	Mental health services linked with primary care, with a focus on education and prevention	Community mental health programs activated and expanded after tsunami·

Table 3.3 Mental health policies and legislation in countries of East and South-East Asia.

		Mental health legislation	
		Present	Absent
Mental health policy or program	Present	Indonesia, Japan, Malaysia, Mongolia, Myanmar, North Korea, Singapore, South Korea, Thailand	Cambodia, China, Laos, Philippines, Viet Nam
	Absent	Brunei	Timor-Leste

Source: [6, 33, 65]; Thailand Mental Health Act (Thailand).

by utilizing political and popular will to reinforce national mental health policies [30].

East and South-East Asia

Mental health legislation and policies are present in relatively more countries of the East and South-East Asia region. Table 3.3 shows the presence of mental health policies and laws in each of the countries in this WHO region; processes to renew policy and laws are underway in South Korea, Japan, and Singapore. Despite 20 years of effort, China does not yet have a national mental health law, though it has instituted a national mental health plan [32], whilst Hong Kong has a mental health ordinance [33]. In Thailand, mental health legislation came into effect in 2008 [34].

Compulsory admission and guardianship

Voluntary and compulsory (involuntary) admissions are regulated by law throughout the region, usually with family involvement. Even in Singapore and Malaysia, where Western influences are somewhat more prevalent, the family plays a major role in the patient's admission and treatment. Involuntary admission with family consent is legalized in Japan and South Korea [35]. China also permits involuntary admission with family consent, although the practice is not legalized, and legal guardians include not only family members but also public officers [36]. Across the region, efforts are being made to ensure that the majority of patients are voluntarily admitted to psychiatric hospitals [37–39].

Community-based mental health care

Legislation has been enacted to support community integration in Japan, Malaysia, Mongolia, and South Korea, whilst most of the other countries in the region have some form of policy which refer to the principle of developing community-based mental health care policies or programs (except for Brunei and Laos) [6].

Australasia and South Pacific

The establishment of recovery-focused, community-oriented services is government policy in both Australia and New Zealand. Both countries have National Mental Health Strategies and Plans. In Australia, each of the states and territories has its own plans, which incorporate elements of the national plan and areas for service development relevant to their jurisdiction.

Australia developed its National Mental Health Strategy in 1992. It comprised four major documents: the National Mental Health Policy, the National Mental Health Plan, the Mental Health Statement of Rights and Responsibilities, and the Medicare Agreements (the latter referring to funding arrangements to support the reform agenda) [40].

The First Australian National Mental Health Plan promoted the integration of inpatient and community services into a cohesive mental health program. Subsequently, there have been three revisions to the original plan. The Second and Third National Mental Health Plans continued in the direction of the original plan, but expanded the focus of reform to include additional activities such as: promotion and prevention to complement the development of the specialist mental health service system; the development of partnerships in service reform, and especially the rights of consumers and their families; and strengthening quality and service responsiveness, fostering research, innovation, and sustainability [40–42].

The Fourth National Mental Health Plan was released in 2009. It takes a more explicit population health approach (heralded in the Third Plan) and seeks to implement the National Mental Health Policy revised by the Coalition of Australian Government Ministers in 2008. The policy is underpinned by eight principles:
- respect for the rights and needs of consumers, carers, and families
- services delivered with a commitment to a recovery approach
- social inclusion
- recognition of social, cultural, and geographic diversity and experience
- recognition that the focus of care may be different across the lifespan
- services delivered to support continuity and coordination of care
- service equity across areas, communities, and age groups
- consideration of the spectrum of mental health, mental health problems, and mental illness.

The Fourth Plan has eight priority areas with a set of measureable indicators, including: social inclusion and recovery; service access, coordination, and continuity of care; prevention and early intervention; quality improvement and innovation; and accountability—measuring and reporting progress. Each of the plans has had a corresponding report on progress, as a vehicle for accountability [43].

Australia also has a set of National Mental Health Standards [44], as well as National Practice Standards for the Mental Health Workforce [45]. The policy field is also informed by other key documents, including Mental Health and Well-being Surveys [46] and the Productivity Commissions Report on Mental Health [47].

New Zealand developed its National Mental Health Strategy "Looking Forward" in 1992. Together with its revision in 1996, "Moving Forward" formed the basis of the first National Mental Health Plan. The second Mental Health Plan ("Te Tahuhu") was released in 2005 [48]. Importantly, it has an explicit combined approach to both mental health and addictions. A series of key challenges for improving mental health and addictions and "delivering meaningful results for people" were defined by the Second Plan, including:

- promotion and prevention
- building mental health and addiction services
- responsiveness
- workforce and culture for recovery
- Maori mental health
- primary health care
- addictions
- funding mechanisms for recovery
- transparency and trust
- working together.

An action plan based on these challenges, "Te Kokiri", was developed and is currently being implemented. "Te Tahuhu" specifies the government's goals for mental health and addictions. In particular, it sets out what all New Zealanders, people with mental illness and/or addictions, and their families and friends should expect from their mental health and addictions services, namely:

- All New Zealanders can see a trusted and high-performing mental health and addictions sector, and have confidence that they are able to access high-quality mental health and addictions services, should they need them.
- People with mental illness and/or addictions are able to experience trustworthy agencies that work across boundaries and enable service users to lead their own recovery. They should experience recovery-focused mental health and addictions services that provide choice, promote independence, and are effective, efficient, responsive, and timely.
- Families and friends are able to experience agencies which operate in a way that enables them to support their family members' recovery and maintain their own well-being.

The Mental Health Commission (established in 1996 to ensure implementation of the National Mental Health Plan and to act as an independent voice for service users and families) developed a national blueprint for the funding of mental health services [49]. Based on a recovery approach, it provided a practical framework for service development. As of 2009 the blueprint has been 80% implemented (MOH, personal communication) and has seen a 154% real increase in the funding of mental health and addiction services.

Like those in Australia, New Zealand has a set of National Mental Health Standards, which have been incorporated in the National Health and Disability Standards [50]. Related key supporting policy documents influencing the development of mental health and addiction services include those relating to Primary Mental Healthcare (PMHC), work-force development [51], a Maori Mental Health Strategy [52], and a National Information Systems Strategy [53].

A variety of programs are offered in both countries addressing mental health promotion, antidiscrimination and destigmatization, prevention, psychiatric treatment, primary mental health care, recovery, and service integration. Despite this, however, considerable unmet needs and continuing government efforts are still found in both countries.

In contrast, mental health policy is less well developed in countries across the Pacific Nations. Policy, planning, and program development in these countries is proceeding in a variety of ways, with different priorities being given to each. However, 14 countries were expected to have a final draft of a mental health policy in place by March 2010 (including the Solomon Islands, Samoa, Papua New Guinea, Guam, and Kiribati), which may provide a firm basis to gain government commitment for the protection of the rights of people with mental illness and, where necessary, also provide a structure for new or updated mental health legislation [37, 54, 55].

Key points in this chapter

- Mental health policies and legislation vary widely within and across regions.
- Whilst some countries have detailed mental health policies and legislation in place, these are often many years, or even decades, old.
- The countries that do have comprehensive and up-to-date mental health policies and legislation in place tend to be those with higher levels of resources.
- It is still uncommon to find a broad statement of national mental health strategy (policies) accompanied by specific implementation plans.

References

[1] Knapp M, McDaid D, Mossialos E, Thornicroft G. Mental Health Policy and Practice Across Europe: An Overview. In: Knapp M, McDaid D, Mossialos E, Thornicroft G, editors. Mental Health Policy and Practice Across Europe. Maidenhead: Open University Press; 2007. pp. 1–14.

[2] World Health Organization. Mental Health Declaration for Europe: Facing the Challenges, Building Solutions. 2005.

[3] World Health Organization. Mental Health Action Plan for Europe: Facing the Challenges, Building Solutions. 2005.

[4] McDaid D, Curran C, Knapp M. Promoting mental well-being in the workplace: a European policy perspective. Int Rev Psychiatry 2005 Oct;17(5):365–73.

[5] World Health Organization. Policies and Practices for Mental Health in Europe: Meeting the Challenges. 2008.

[6] World Health Organization. Mental Health Atlas, revised edition. 2005.

[7] Semrau M, Barley E, Law A, Thornicroft G. Lessons learned in developing community mental health care (3): Europe. World Psychiatry; 2011 (in press).

[8] Thornicroft G, Rose D. Mental health in Europe. British Medical Journal 2005;330(7492):613–14.

[9] Knapp MJ, McDaid D, Mossialos E, Thornicroft G. Mental Health Policy and Practice Across Europe. Buckingham: Open University Press; 2007.

[10] World Health Organization. WHO-AIMS Report on Mental Health System in the Republic of Azerbaijan Baku, Azerbaijan: WHO and Ministry of Health. 2007.

[11] WHO-AIMS Report on Mental Health System in the Kyrgyz Republic Bishkek, Kyrgyz Republic: WHO and Ministry of Health. 2008.

[12] World Health Organization. European Health for All Database. 2009.

[13] World Health Organization. WHO-AIMS Report on Mental Health System in Armenia Yerevan, Armenia: WHO and Ministry of Health. 2009.

[14] Alarcon RD, Aguilar-Gaxiola SA. Mental health policy developments in Latin America. Bulletin of the World Health Organization 2000;78(4):483–90.

[15] Almeida JM. Estrategias de cooperación técnica de la Organización Panamericana de la Salud en la nueva fase de la reforma de los servicios de salud mental en América Latina y el Caribe. Revista Panamericana de Salud Pública 2005;18(4/5):314–26.

[16] Levav I, Restrepo H, Guerra de MC. The restructuring of psychiatric care in Latin America: a new policy for mental health services. J Public Health Policy 1994;15(1):71–85.

[17] Mari JJ, Saraceno B, Rodriguez J, Levav I. Mental health systems in Latin America and Caribbean countries: a change in the making. Psychol Med 2007 Oct;37(10):1514–16.

[18] Razzouk D, Gregorio G, Antunes R, Mari J. Lessons learned in developing community mental health care (5): Latin American and Caribbean Countries. World Psychiatry; 2011 (in press).

[19] Institute of Medicine. Mental, Neurological, and Substance Use Disorders in Sub-Saharan Africa: Reducing the Treatment Gap, Increasing Quality of Care: Workshop Summary. Washington DC: Institute of Medicine; 2010.

[20] Jenkins R, Baingana F, Belkin G, Borowitz M, Daly A, Francis P, et al. Mental health and the development agenda in Sub-Saharan Africa. Psychiatr Serv 2010 Mar;61(3):229–34.

[21] Gureje O. The WPA Regional Meeting in Abuja, Nigeria,22–24 October 2009. World Psychiatry 2010 Feb;9(1):63–4.

[22] Gureje O, Jenkins R. Mental health in development: re-emphasising the link. Lancet 2007 Feb 10;369(9560):447–9.

[23] Flisher AJ, Lund C, Funk M, Banda M, Bhana A, Doku V, et al. Mental health policy development and implementation in four African countries. J Health Psychol 2007 May;12(3):505–16.

[24] Draper CE, Lund C, Kleintjes S, Funk M, Omar M, Flisher AJ. Mental health policy in South Africa: development process and content. Health Policy Plan 2009 Sep;24(5):342–56.

[25] Lund C. Mental health in Africa: Findings from the Mental Health and Poverty Project. Int Rev Psychiatry 2010;22(6):547–9.

[26] Bird P, Omar M, Doku V, Lund C, Nsereko JR, Mwanza J. Increasing the priority of mental health in Africa: findings from qualitative research in Ghana, South Africa, Uganda and Zambia. Health Policy Plan; 2010 Dec 8.

[27] Lund C. Mental Health Policy Implementation in Ghana and in Zambia. Afr J Psychiatry (Johannesbg) 2010 Jul;13(3):165–7.

[28] Omar MA, Green AT, Bird PK, Mirzoev T, Flisher AJ, Kigozi F, et al. Mental health policy process: a comparative study of Ghana, South Africa, Uganda and Zambia. Int J Ment Health Syst 2010;4:24.

[29] Trivedi JK, Goel D, Kallivayalil RA, Isaac M, Shrestha DM, Gambheera HC. Regional cooperation in South Asia in the field of mental health. World Psychiatry 2007;6:57–9.

[30] Trivedi JK, Narang P, Dhyani M. Mental health legislation in South Asia with special reference to India: shortcomings and solutions. Mental Health Review Journal 2007;12(3):22–29.

[31] Patel V, Prince M. Global mental health: a new global health field comes of age. JAMA 2010 May 19;303(19):1976–7.

[32] Asia-Australia Mental Health (AAMH). Summary Report: Asia-Pacific Community Mental Health Development Project. 2008.

[33] Editorial. What we should consider when we next amend the mental health ordinance of Hong Kong. The Hong Kong Journal of Psychiatry 2009;19:53–6.

[34] Thailand Mental Health Act. Thailand Mental Health Act, BE2008. 2010.

[35] Lee MS, Hoe M, Hwang TY, Lee YM. Service priority and standard performance of community mental health centers in South Korea: A Delphi approach. Psychiatry Investigation 2009;6:59–65.

[36] Kokai M. China. In: Shinfuku N, Asai K, editors. Mental Health in the World, revised edition. Tokyo: Health Press; 2009. pp. 131–7.

[37] Deva MP. Psychosocial rehabilitation models in the Asia-Pacific region. Psychiatry Clin Neurosci 1998 Dec;52 Suppl: S364–S366.

[38] Ito H, Setoya Y, Suzuki Y. Lessons learned in developing community mental health care. 7: East and Southeast Asia. World Psychiatry; 2011 (in press).

[39] Saxena S, Sharan P, Saraceno B. Budget and financing of mental health services: baseline information on 89 countries from WHO's project atlas. J Ment Health Policy Econ 2003 Sep;6(3):135–43.

[40] Department of Health and Aging. National Mental Health Report: Summary of 15 years of reform. Canberra: Commonwealth of Australia; 2010.

[41] Meadows G. Mental Health Services in Australia. In: Meadows G, Singh B, Grigg M, editors. Mental Health in Australia, 2nd edition. Melbourne: Oxford University Press; 2008. pp. 69–75.

[42] Betts V, Thornicroft G. International Mid-Term Review of the Second National Mental Health Plan for Australia. Canberra: Commonwealth of Australia; 2001.

[43] Department of Health and Aging. National Mental Health Report: Summary of 15 years of reform. Canberra: Commonwealth of Australia; 2010.

[44] Department of Health and Aging (DOHA). National Standards for Mental Health Services. Canberra: Commonwealth of Australia; 2010.

[45] Department of Health and Aging. National Practice Standards for the Mental Health Workforce. Canberra: Commonwealth of Australia; 2002.

[46] Australian Bureau of Statistics (ABS). National Survey of Mental Health and Well-being. 2007.

[47] Australian Government Productivity Commission. Australia's Health Workforce: Productivity Commission Research Report. Melbourne: Australian Government Productivity Commission; 2005.

[48] Ministry of Health. Te Tahuhu: Improving Mental Health 2005–2015. The Second New Zealand Mental Health and Addiction Plan. 2005.

[49] Mental Health Commission. Blueprint for Mental Health Services in New Zealand. 1998. NZ, Mental Health Commission.

[50] Ministry of Health. Health and Disability Service Standards. 2008. Ministry of Health.

[51] Ministry of Health. Tauawhitia te Wero: Embracing the Challenge: National mental health and addiction workforce development plan 2006–2009. Ministry of Health; 2005.

[52] Ministry of Health. Te Puawaiwhero: The second Maori mental health and addiction national strategic framework 2008–2015. Ministry of Health; 2008.

[53] Ministry of Health. National Mental Health Information Strategy 2005–2010. Ministry of Health; 2005.

[54] McGeorge P. Lessons learned in developing community mental health care (2): Australasia and the South Pacific. World Psychiatry; 2011 (in press).

[55] Asia-Australia Mental Health (AAMH). Summary Report: Asia-Pacific Community Mental Health Development Project. 2008.

[56] World Health Organization. WHO-AIMS report on mental health system in Afghanistan. Kabul: World Health Organization; 2006.

[57] World Health Organization. WHO-AIMS report on mental health system in Bangladesh. Dhaka: World Health Organization; 2007.

[58] World Health Organization. WHO-AIMS report on mental health system in Bhutan. Thimpu: World Health Organization; 2006.

[59] Nagaraja D, Murthy P. Mental health care and human rights. New Delhi and Bangalore: National Human Rights Commission and National Institute of Mental Health and Neurosciences; 2008.

[60] Murthy SR. The national mental health programme: progress and problems. In: Agarwal SP, Goel DS editors. New Delhi: Directorate General of Health Services, Ministry of Health and Family Welfare; 2004. pp. 75–91.

[61] World Health Organization. WHO-AIMS report on mental health system in Maldives. Male: World Health Organization; 2006.

[62] World Health Organization. WHO-AIMS report on mental health system in Nepal. Kathmandu: World Health Organization; 2009.

[63] World Health Organization. WHO-AIMS Report On Mental Health System in Pakistan. Karachi: World Health Organization; 2009.

[64] WHO Country Office for Sri Lanka. Mental health update. Colombo: World Health Organization; 2008.

[65] Jacob KS, Sharan P, Mirza I, Garrido-Cumbrera M, Seedat S, Mari JJ, et al. Mental health systems in countries: Where are we now? Lancet 2007;370(9592):1061–77.

Implementation of community mental health services

CHAPTER 4

The current provision of community mental health services

Introduction

This chapter provides an overview of the community mental health services developed within each of the seven regions. Each region is discussed in turn.

Africa

In most African countries, specialized psychiatric hospitals are still the mainstay of treatment for the mentally ill, and only 57% of African countries have reported having community-based mental health care [1]. In the light of mental health reforms occurring across the world, there has been a move by some African countries to decentralize specialist mental health services, opening outpatient facilities and, in some places, inpatient beds within general hospitals. However, the level of integration of mental health is limited in most instances, and often specialist mental health services are isolated from general health services in terms of both staff and administration.

The majority of countries (83%) in the Africa region claim to have mental health care integrated into primary health care services [2]. However, what is actually meant by this is not clear. Only 61% of countries provide evidence that there is actual treatment of mental health problems in primary health care, and an even lower proportion of countries (59%) report that primary health care workers are trained in mental health care. There is substantial heterogeneity across the region in terms of the personnel available in the primary health care setting (e.g. ranging from mental health nurses and medical doctors in South Africa, to health officers, general nurses, and health extension workers (HEWs) in Ethiopia). There is

Community Mental Health: putting policy into practice globally, First Edition. Graham Thornicroft, Maya Semrau, Atalay Alem, Robert E. Drake, Hiroto Ito, Jair Mari, Peter McGeorge, and R. Thara. © 2011 John Wiley & Sons, Ltd. Published 2011 by John Wiley & Sons, Ltd.

also variability in what is understood by "mental health care in primary health care". In some countries primary mental health care is conceptualized as the treatment of patients by mental health workers in a primary health care setting, or follow-up of patients discharged from inpatient psychiatric care (e.g. Mauritius); for others it means psychiatric outpatient follow-up located at a health center (Seychelles); and for some it is the ability of primary health care workers to diagnose and treat the majority of cases, with referral of more complex cases.

Despite recommendations by the World Health Organization (WHO) and others [3], there are only a few examples of specialist mental health workers being utilized to support mental health in primary health care through coordination and planning of local mental health care, supervision, in-service training, consultation for complex cases, and prevention and promotion activities. Indeed, only one of the Africa regional experts consulted in our expert survey (see Chapter 1 for details) considered expansion of prevention and promotion activities to be an aim for developing community mental health care.

Although more holistic care is an expected benefit of community mental health services, especially when integrated into the primary health care system, as our review has identified (see Chapter 1 for details), studies have not necessarily shown this to be occurring [4, 5]. Time pressures, a strongly biomedical model of care, and limited resources to support non-medication interventions may mean that mental health care is reduced to the dispensing and administration of medication [6].

In the absence of provision for rehabilitation, residential facilities for those who are severely disabled by mental health problems, and day center facilities, some commentators have argued that a community-based model of mental health care may not be workable in under-resourced settings, with the potential to exacerbate disadvantage, neglect, and exclusion [7]. Some support for this came from both patients and their families in South Africa, who expressed a preference for long-stay hospital care rather than community-based follow-up [8,9]. Innovative solutions have been piloted, largely drawing on existing community resources—for example rehabilitation villages in Tanzania [10] and Nigeria [11]—although questions remain about their sustainability and generalizability [12]. Public–private partnerships, most often between governmental services and nongovernmental organizations (NGOs), have been suggested as one way to meet needs [13], for example through setting up income-generating activities [14].

Without community sensitization and engagement, the detection of untreated patients and take-up of mental health care is unlikely to proceed successfully. Similarly, without strategies in place to deal with patients who default from care, mental health care in primary health care may not be sufficiently flexible to respond to the particular needs of patients with mental health difficulties. As more specialist mental health workers tend to be located at regional and district levels of the health system in most African countries, they are limited in their ability to provide responsive outreach services close to home. A number of countries have made use of trained community-based volunteers to overcome this problem [14, 15], but the difficulty of maintaining motivation and sustaining the system when workers are not remunerated has been highlighted [16]. One opportunity for the future might be use of a new cadre of paid primary health care workers being introduced into some African countries, such as Ethiopia: the HEWs. The remit of HEWs is to visit all homes in their catchment area on a regular basis, with a focus on providing preventive and promotive care. In Ethiopia, HEWs are now being trained in the detection of persons with mental illness. Use of service-user groups to help support community outreach services has also been applied successfully [14].

The potential role of traditional healers and religious leaders in the delivery of community-based care has been much discussed [17, 18], but with few examples of this happening in practice. As traditional healers have been the main providers of mental health care in many African countries, scaling up integration of mental health into primary health care without considering the place of traditional healing could possibly run the risk of alienating individuals from their communities. One example of traditional healers providing counseling services in conjunction with a community-based mental health service has been reported, although with no evaluation of patient outcomes [14].

The potential contribution of support groups, composed of service users and care givers, to improving clinical outcomes and social inclusion, as well as lobbying for improved services, has been described but not formally evaluated [19, 20].

Australasia and South Pacific

Mental health services in Australia and New Zealand have influenced each other's development and as a consequence have developed along similar lines in terms of models of service delivery. Some Australian jurisdictions, however (such as Victoria), have more in common with developments in New Zealand than others. Pacific Nations, by comparison, are at a rudimentary stage of development and are only just beginning to set in place processes that may begin to adequately address the needs of their people with mental illnesses.

Funding and governance
Services in Australasia are funded and governed differently in the two countries, which has led to varying degrees and types of progress in their

service development. In Australia, the federal (Commonwealth) government has a benefit system (Medicare) in place, supporting access of the
general public to treatment by general practitioners and psychiatrists, psychologists, and other mental health professionals working in private practice. Health insurance firms also play a significant role in the funding of
private mental health practitioners. In addition, NGOs are supported by
federal agencies such as the Department of Families, Housing, Community Services and Indigenous Affairs (FaHCSIA), though they also obtain
their funding from a variety of other sources, including state government
departments.

Responsibility for the governance and management of public mental
health services has traditionally been assigned to the individual states
and territories through their government departments of health, and a
system of area and sector health services providing services for populations between 1 and 2 million. Health services are currently being
reorganized to achieve greater coordination between federal and state governments. However, the prevailing federal and state/territories system has
been severely criticized as being responsible for a lack of integration between federal and state government mental health initiatives, and despite
obvious gains as one of the reasons for a lack of progress in implementing
the National Mental Health Plan (1992) (see Chapter 3 for details of this
plan).

Whilst the situation is changing, 8.3% of mental health funding in
Australia is allocated to NGOs [21], compared with New Zealand where
30% of mental health funding is assigned to NGOs. By contrast, under
a series of initiatives sponsored by the Council of Australian Governments, Australia funds primary health care to a much greater extent than
New Zealand, with this funding at latest estimates amounting to 339 million AUD (372 million USD), compared to 24 million NZD (19 million
USD) in New Zealand.

In New Zealand there is a funder/provider split in health services. Whilst
some NGO funding is provided through sources other than health departments, most funding for both public mental health services and NGOs is
delivered through 21 district health boards (DHBs). In addition, a much
smaller amount continues to be allocated on a national basis through the
Ministry of Health. Overall, this system allows for a more coherent system
of funding than in Australia, and is based largely on the delivery of public
rather than private services, though NGOs do compete with one another
and (in theory) with specialist clinical services for service contracts.

New Zealand also has a Mental Health Commission, which since 1998
has monitored how services are functioning and the progress in the
implementation of the National Mental Health Plan. It is also charged
with supporting service improvements and the reduction of stigma and

discrimination against people with mental illnesses and/or addictions. The Commission's "Mental Health Blueprint—How Things Should Be" [22], which specified the services and staffing that should be in place for populations of 100 000, is now being superseded by more contemporary funding frameworks. However, it has been hugely instrumental in holding services to account and in guiding decision-making by funders and providers alike over the course of the past decade.

The Pacific Nations' health services are generally publicly funded through departments of health, although spending on mental health remains minimal and in some cases cannot be identified separately from other health spending. NGOs are also publicly funded, though some are privately financed through their own international organizations. In some of the larger nations (such as Guam, New Caledonia, and Northern Marianas) funding is also available through a mixture of private and social insurance systems.

Service provision

Both Australia and New Zealand have a mix of local and regional, public and private mental health services. The private system in New Zealand is not government subsidized and as a consequence is insignificant compared to that of Australia.

Services cover children and adolescents, general adults, and the elderly, with priority having been given to the seriously mentally ill in the development of community mental health services in both Australia and New Zealand. That said, treatments for high-prevalence disorders are now receiving increasing emphasis through primary mental health care initiatives established over the past decade. Whilst significant service gaps remain in some areas and many services are still not adequately integrated [23], overall across the two countries a comprehensive mix of hospital- and community-based services has been established (see Table 4.1).

Table 4.1 Range of mental health services available in Australasia and the South Pacific.

Service	Australia	New Zealand	South Pacific
Primary health care	+	+/−	+
Outpatient/ambulatory clinics	+	+	+/−
Community mental health teams	+	+	−
Acute inpatient care	+	+	+/−
Long-term residential care in the community	+	+	−
Rehabilitation, work, occupation	+	+	+/−

Legend: + present, +/− variable, − absent

Based on Thornicroft and Tansella's categorization of mental health services [24] (and including provision through primary health care), Australian and New Zealander consumers have potential access to all service categories specified in the framework outlined in Table 4.1 (though services are not available in all areas, or to everybody who may need them). It is important to note that in both Australia and New Zealand (particularly the latter), most of the services included in Table 4.1 have been further differentiated in terms of specialization, providers, and target groups. Specialist community services, for example, supported in some cases by residential programs, have been established to provide care for people with specific disorders and circumstances, including:
- forensic psychiatry
- maternal mental health
- peer support services
- early psychosis
- cultural services (particularly in New Zealand with the establishment of Maori and Pacific Island mental health services)
- homelessness
- eating disorders
- addictions, ranging from alcohol and drugs to problems with gambling and Internet addictions
- post-traumatic stress disorder, covering sexual abuse and family violence
- affective disorders
- anxiety disorders.

Some of these, such as forensic psychiatry and early psychosis services, despite branding as "Cinderella" (i.e. less favored) services, have become major modes of service delivery in their own right, much to the chagrin of those generalist services with which they interface, such as general adult services, and in the latter case child and adolescent services. There is now also a range of providers, from primary health care clinicians to NGO and peer (service-user) workers, providing services for people that would otherwise have been the exclusive domain of specialist clinicians.

Whilst many rural areas have similar service and staffing issues to those of low- or middle-income countries (LAMICs), most medium to large urban areas have a full range of clinical and nonclinical mental health staff employed in services, and are developing new occupational classes of workers. Support for rural areas is often provided by larger urban services and visiting practitioners.

It is important to note that within Australia and New Zealand progress in implementing National Mental Health Plan targets (see Chapter 3) shows significant jurisdictional and regional variations. In Australia, these variations are not straightforward, with some jurisdictions such as Western Australia employing above-average clinical staff in ambulatory care whilst at the same time funding NGOs much less than other regions. The Australian Capital Territory appears to have made the most progress in terms of ambulatory clinical staff and funding to NGOs, as well as the number of staffed community residential beds and the relatively low number of inpatient beds. By contrast, New South Wales has made poor progress on all these indicators. Victoria, long regarded as the paragon for community care in Australia, now falls somewhere between these jurisdictions [21]. In New Zealand, whilst there are regional variations, the smaller size of the country, a more coherent health system, and arguably a greater commitment to community care, have all resulted in more homogeneity in the implementation of community care than in Australia.

In Australia and New Zealand most acute services are now provided through community-based services (public, not for profit, private, and primary health care), supported by acute inpatient services provided in general and private hospitals (the latter being insignificant in New Zealand). Innovation of services such as home-based treatment, crisis respite, and peer-run acute services (such as those implemented by the Counties Manukau District Health Board in New Zealand) are gathering momentum. However, such innovation is competing with an increasing emphasis on relocating community teams to hospital bases and the exponential growth of mental health care delivered by emergency departments in general hospitals. Care for people with longer-term disorders is provided mainly in the community by public continuing-care mental health teams and NGOs. There are also inpatient rehabilitation and forensic services provided through the public sector in both countries (which in Australia are assuming increasing significance in the overall continuum of care).

In both Australia and New Zealand an increasing and organized focus on services for people with high-prevalence disorders has been taking place over the past decade, with more attention and funding being given to the delivery of services involving primary health care, and in the case of Australia private psychiatry and psychology practices. Additional services for the treatment of people with mild to moderate disorders are occurring through the delivery of Web-based programs funded in the main by government and university agencies. The range of specialized programs such as early psychosis, maternal mental health, peer support, and alcohol and drug services is largely provided by community-based agencies including public and private mental health services and NGOs.

Criticism continues to be directed, by some observers, at health authorities in Australia for addressing problems with a return to a focus on hospital-based care delivered through emergency departments and intensive acute and rehabilitation inpatient units. Although the Council of Australian Ministers has developed and is implementing through the jurisdictions an "Action Plan", criticisms of the IV National Mental Health Plan have focused on the lack of detail required to implement practical initiatives to improve the landscape of services available to the public [28].

In New Zealand, whilst noting the extensive range of examples of innovative funding and services, the Mental Health Commission in its ongoing monitoring of services delivered by DHBs is aware of similar problems to those identified above. These include problems with accessing acute services, continuity of care, and inadequate levels of community options and support, such as alcohol and drug services for youth and crisis respite care for service users and their families. An apparent drive to continue the shift to community care has received recent government attention through its desire to change the focus of some secondary mental health services to primary health care. However, combined with concerns raised about reductions in NGO funding, questions have been raised about the extent to which the changes are actually being driven by a desire to reduce mental health expenditure overall, rather than a continuing emphasis on the implementation of the National Mental Health Plan and in particular community care.

By contrast, as shown in Table 4.1, mental health services in Pacific Nations are significantly underdeveloped compared with Australia and New Zealand. Services are delivered mainly through village- or community-based primary health care clinics, linked in some cases to regional clinics or national hospitals. In higher-population nations, such as Fiji and Papua New Guinea, inpatient units are also available, but, more often than not, the care they provide is not particularly differentiated in terms of specific disorders. Moreover, some inpatient units remain unused because of concerns about safety and/or insufficient staff to manage patients in need of inpatient care. As a result, some people with serious mental illnesses are detained in police custody, without access to appropriate treatment [25].

It is difficult to estimate the proportion of community mental health services compared with inpatient care in Pacific Island Nations. Indeed, it is questionable how meaningful this would be given the challenges of their current state of development. Mental illness is still not widely accepted as a concept by much of the population, and resources dedicated to it are meager at best. We do know, however, that "most middle- and low-income countries have not increased their expenditure on mental health services by much more than 1% of their health expenditure to mental health" [26]. In addition, mental health initiatives do not readily attract sponsorship from private or corporate donors, particularly in view of the long-term commitment that this requires. The reality is then that underfunding, disinterest, and prejudice against people with mental illnesses continue to result in their neglect, mistreatment, and marginalization.

Fully trained mental health clinicians are employed in some nations, though not in anywhere near sufficient numbers to address need. Pacific Nations rely instead on generally trained health professionals (often nurses), NGOs, and other workers such as "traditional healers" who are engaged to assist in the care of people with mental illnesses and addictions. There are few permanently based psychiatrists serving the region; however, this situation is ameliorated to some extent by the employment of visiting psychiatrists from Australia and New Zealand, and in some cases the USA.

In the Pacific Island Nations considerable progress has been made by the 18 pilot-member countries of the Pacific Islands Mental Health Network (PIMHnet) in recent years. PIMHnet is a joint initiative of the WHO Regional Office for the Western Pacific and the WHO Headquarters in Geneva (see Chapter 5 for further details). PIMHnet has supported the building of infrastructures that are supportive to services within individual countries, and decreases reliance on external measures such as visiting clinicians. Measures to improve infrastructure include the development of local training initiatives for primary health workers (including designing or adapting assessment tools for local use) and the provision of mentoring and support services within and between countries, using technological tools such as telehealth. A recent review of PIMHnet, undertaken for NZAID, concluded, "The findings of the review suggest that a very successful project has been implemented and the interventions so far have been implemented well, measured at this early stage primarily in outputs delivered. The achievements are significant given the short period of time that the project has been in place and the number of countries that are now benefiting" [27].

Europe

Generally, a wider range of community mental health services exist within Europe than within most other regions worldwide, with at least some service components available in every country in the region (in comparison, in 2005 about 68% of countries worldwide had community mental health services, with around 83% of the population worldwide covered [2]). However, whilst a few countries lead the way in the successful implementation of community-based mental health services according to an evidence-based "Balanced Care Model" that integrates elements of community and hospital services [24,29–32], in many others access to community-based services is still very limited and may commonly consist of small pilot projects [33].

Broadly speaking, consistent with economic differences across the region, the division is mostly between the Eastern and Western countries of Europe. In the EU-15 countries and other predominantly Western high-income countries, following a move towards human rights, social inclusion, and empowerment over the last few decades, a large array of multidisciplinary community-based services may be available to people with mental health problems, with most patients being treated outside of mental institutions [34]. In line with the Balanced Care Model approach, the mental hospitals that do exist in these countries are often relatively small, close to communities [33], and usually located in acute wards in general hospitals, with hospital stays reduced as far as possible [31, 35].

In the low- or lower middle-income non-EU countries of Eastern Europe, in particular the CIS countries, access to community-based care tends to be far more limited. Large mental health institutions are commonly still the mainstay of the mental health care system [34], and community mental health services are often restricted to polyclinics or dispensaries attached to a psychiatric office. Where any additional community-based services exist, these are often implemented by NGOs or international agencies. The range and quality of mental health services in the post-2004 EU countries and other middle-income countries tends to lie somewhere between those of the EU-15 and CIS countries. However, the boundaries of this divide are blurry, and no two countries in the region have the exact same mental health system in place.

Inpatient services

In general, the number of psychiatric beds has been decreasing steadily across Europe and mental hospitals are increasingly being closed down [36]. However, in some countries this process has been much slower than in others [34, 35]. Although inpatient services in mental hospitals still exist in almost all European countries (the exceptions are Italy, Iceland, Andorra, Monaco, and San Marino), the number of psychiatric beds and the balance between beds in mental institutions and inpatient community-based facilities varies greatly between countries (see Table 4.2). Also, whilst in some countries the small or absent number of inpatient beds is due to the substantial progress that has been made in replacing mental hospitals with community-based care (in the UK and Italy for example), in others (such as Albania and Turkey) the small number of beds reflects a lack in funding and a deficit in service provision for mental health overall. Other countries, primarily EU-15 countries such as Belgium, France, Germany, and the Netherlands, have a combination of large numbers of inpatient beds and community services [33]. However, in most European countries (in particular those in Eastern parts) institutional care still outweighs community care by far, with around two-thirds of all psychiatric beds across the region still located in mental hospitals [36].

Table 4.2 Overview of mental health inpatient services across the European region.

	Mental hospitals (inpatient services)	Community psychiatric inpatient units/units in district general hospitals	Total number of psychiatric beds per 100 000 population	Percentage of psychiatric beds in facilities other than mental hospitals (approximate)
Former EU-15				
Austria	Yes	Yes	52	29%
Belgium	Yes	Yes	152	42%
Denmark	Yes	Yes	61	N/A
Finland	Yes	Yes	72	99%
France	Yes	Yes	95	42%
Germany	Yes	Yes	75	40%
Greece	Yes	Yes	18	22%
Ireland	Yes	Yes	94	24%
Italy	No	Yes	8	100%
Luxembourg	Yes	Yes	97	46%
Netherlands	Yes	Yes	114	18%
Portugal	Yes	Yes	27	37%
Spain	Yes	Yes	47	16%
Sweden	Yes	Yes	54	93%
United Kingdom	Yes	Yes	23	39%
Other EU				
Bulgaria	Yes	Yes	64	56%
Cyprus	Yes	Yes	27	22%
Czech Republic	Yes	Yes	110	13%
Estonia	Yes	Yes	56	22%
Hungary	Yes	Yes	93	76%
Latvia	Yes	Yes	148	7%
Lithuania	Yes	Yes	88	11%
Malta	Yes	Yes	185	under 1%
Poland	Yes	Yes	65	25%
Romania	Yes	Yes	75	28%
Slovakia	Yes	Yes	96	81%
Slovenia	Yes	Yes	85	15%
South-Eastern				
Albania	Yes	Yes	24	25%
Bosnia and Herzegovina	Yes	Yes	36	33%
Croatia	Yes	Yes	93	20%
Georgia	Yes	No	29	0%
Montenegro	Yes	No	49	0%
Serbia	Yes	Yes	95	N/A
T.F.Y.R. of Macedonia	Yes	Yes	74	14%
Turkey	Yes	Yes	12	25%

(Continued)

Table 4.2 Continued.

	Mental hospitals (inpatient services)	Community psychiatric inpatient units/units in district general hospitals	Total number of psychiatric beds per 100 000 population	Percentage of psychiatric beds in facilities other than mental hospitals (approximate)
CIS				
Armenia	Yes	Yes	45	under 1%
Azerbaijan	Yes	No	48	0%
Belarus	Yes	Yes	70	6%
Kazakhstan	Yes	Yes	63	9%
Kyrgyzstan	Yes	Yes	43	10%
Republic of Moldova	Yes	No	63	0%
Russian Federation	Yes	Yes	112	12%
Tajikistan	Yes	N/A	25	N/A
Turkmenistan	Yes	Yes	33	9%
Ukraine	Yes	Yes	94	3%
Uzbekistan	Yes	Yes	32	3%
Other				
Andorra	No	Yes	15	100%
Iceland	No	Yes	50	100%
Israel	Yes	Yes	59	7%
Monaco	No	Yes	173	100%
Norway	Yes	Yes	119	42%
San Marino	No	Yes	38	100%
Switzerland	Yes	Yes	106	6%

N/A: information not available.
Data taken from WHO publications [2, 33, 37, 39,126, 127]. Where data were conflicting between publications, the most recent source was used.

Mental health in primary health care

Whilst all countries in the European region increasingly have mental health services integrated into primary health care (see Table 4.3), and generally the role of primary health care for people with mental health problems has been increasing throughout the region [33], the extent of this varies widely. Whilst all countries in the region for which data exist report that mental health problems may be identified and referrals made to specialist services in primary health care for both common mental disorders (CMDs) and severe mental disorders (SMDs) (apart from Israel for the latter), diagnosis and treatment of mental health problems in primary health care, in particular SMDs, is far less common (see Table 4.3).

Table 4.3 Overview of primary care services for mental health across the European region.

	Mental health in primary health care	Identification and referral to specialist services for CMDs	Diagnosis for CMDs	Treatment of CMDs	Identification and referral to specialist services for SMDs	Diagnosis for SMDs	Treatment of SMDs
Former EU-15							
Austria	Yes	Yes	Yes	Yes	Yes	Yes	Yes
Belgium	Yes	Yes	Yes	Yes	Yes	Yes	Yes
Denmark	Yes	Yes	Yes	Yes	Yes	Yes	Yes
Finland	Yes	Yes	Yes	Yes	Yes	No	Yes
France	Yes	Yes	Yes	Yes	Yes	Yes	Yes
Germany	Yes	Yes	Yes	Yes	Yes	Yes	Yes
Greece	Yes	Yes	N/A	Yes	Yes	N/A	Yes
Ireland	Yes	Yes	Yes	Yes	Yes	Yes	Yes
Italy	Yes	Yes	Yes	Yes	Yes	No	No
Luxembourg	Yes	Yes	Yes	Yes	Yes	Yes	Yes
Netherlands	Yes	Yes	Yes	Yes	Yes	Yes	Yes
Portugal	Yes	Yes	Yes	Yes	Yes	No	No
Spain	Yes	Yes	Yes	Yes	Yes	Yes	Yes
Sweden	Yes	Yes	Yes	Yes	Yes	Yes	Yes
United Kingdom	Yes	Yes	Yes	Yes	Yes	Yes	Yes
Other EU							
Bulgaria	Yes	Yes	Yes	Yes	Yes	Yes	No
Cyprus	Yes	N/A	N/A	N/A	N/A	Yes	Yes
Czech Republic	Yes	Yes	Yes	No	Yes	No	No
Estonia	Yes	Yes	Yes	Yes	Yes	Yes	Yes
Hungary	Yes	Yes	No	Yes	Yes	No	No
Latvia	Yes	Yes	Yes	Yes	Yes	No	No
Lithuania	Yes	Yes	Yes	Yes	Yes	Yes	No
Malta	Yes	Yes	Yes	Yes	Yes	N/A	Yes
Poland	Yes	Yes	Yes	Yes	Yes	Yes	No
Romania	Yes	Yes	Yes	Yes	Yes	No	No
Slovakia	Yes	Yes	Yes	Yes	N/A	N/A	Yes
Slovenia	Yes	N/A	Yes	Yes	Yes	N/A	Yes
South-Eastern							
Albania	Yes	Yes	Yes	Yes	Yes	No	No
Bosnia and Herzegovina	Yes	Yes	Yes	Yes	Yes	No	No
Croatia	Yes	Yes	Yes	Yes	Yes	Yes	No

(Continued)

Table 4.3 Continued.

	Mental health in primary health care	Identification and referral to specialist services for CMDs	Diagnosis for CMDs	Treatment of CMDs	Identification and referral to specialist services for SMDs	Diagnosis for SMDs	Treatment of SMDs
Georgia	Yes	Yes	No	No	Yes	No	No
Montenegro	Yes	Yes	Yes	Yes	Yes	Yes	No
Serbia	Yes	Yes	Yes	Yes	Yes	Yes	No
T.F.Y.R. of Macedonia	Yes	Yes	Yes	No	Yes	No	No
Turkey	Yes	Yes	Yes	Yes	Yes	No	No
CIS							
Armenia	Yes	N/A	N/A	N/A	N/A	N/A	No
Azerbaijan	Yes	Yes	No	No	Yes	No	No
Belarus	Yes	N/A	N/A	N/A	N/A	N/A	Yes
Kazakhstan	Yes	N/A	N/A	N/A	N/A	N/A	No
Kyrgyzstan	Yes	N/A	N/A	N/A	N/A	N/A	No
Republic of Moldova	Yes	Yes	No	Yes	Yes	No	No
Russian Federation	Yes	Yes	Yes	Yes	Yes	No	No
Tajikistan	Yes	N/A	N/A	N/A	N/A	N/A	No
Turkmenistan	Yes	N/A	N/A	N/A	N/A	N/A	No
Ukraine	Yes	N/A	N/A	N/A	N/A	N/A	No
Uzbekistan	Yes	Yes	Yes	No	Yes	Yes	No
Other							
Andorra	Yes	N/A	N/A	N/A	N/A	N/A	Yes
Iceland	Yes	N/A	N/A	N/A	N/A	N/A	Yes
Israel	Yes	Yes	Yes	Yes	No	No	No
Monaco	Yes	N/A	N/A	N/A	N/A	N/A	Yes
Norway	Yes	Yes	Yes	Yes	Yes	Yes	Yes
San Marino	Yes	N/A	N/A	N/A	N/A	N/A	Yes
Switzerland	Yes	Yes	Yes	Yes	Yes	Yes	Yes

N/A: information not available.
Data taken from WHO publications [2, 33, 37, 39,126, 127]. Where data were conflicting between publications, the most recent source was used.

Furthermore, even where mental health services have been integrated into primary health care, these may be integrated poorly. In many countries the primary health care system for mental health is still inadequate [33] or almost lacking (e.g. Armenia [37]), and even in high-income countries the provision of mental health services within primary care has often been found to be less than optimal [38]. Mental health training for primary care staff is only available in around two-thirds of countries [33], and is often insufficient, which frequently results in mental health problems not being recognized or treatment methods being unknown [35, 36].

Community mental health services

Thus, although there is a definite trend towards an increase in community-based mental health services and a decrease in institutional care [33], the pace and scale at which this is occurring, as well the quality of services, varies widely throughout the European region [34, 36]. For instance, at least 85% of countries in the region now report having mental health day care, but in some countries such services tend to be attached to long-term mental hospitals or may be very limited in number, whilst in others there may be a variety of day-care services available in a selection of community settings [33]. Similarly, whilst almost all countries in the region report having outpatient and ambulatory services, there are great disparities in these services across countries. Whilst in EU countries outpatient services are commonly run by a multidisciplinary team in mental hospitals, district general hospitals, or community facilities, with many types of interventions being available in a number of different settings, in many of the Eastern countries these services are usually in form of polyclinics or dispensaries in a larger general clinic run by a psychiatrist. Here there are typically very few support staff and medication is often the only available treatment [33], though in some cases patients may also be followed up in the community [39].

Moreover, access to such services may be very limited within countries, especially in the Eastern parts of the region [33]. Variables such as location, age, gender, ethnicity, employment status, type of diagnosis, educational background, and socioeconomic status may determine whether care, and what type of care, is received [33, 35, 36, 40, 41]. One example of this is that more services tend to be available in urban areas compared to rural settings.

North America

In spite of their geographical proximity and common language (the province of Québec excepted), the USA and Canada have distinct cultures and significantly different health care systems. These differences extend to the organization of community mental health care. Accordingly, we describe community mental health care separately for each country.

The USA

The USA has numerous mental health systems, independent agencies, and single providers. A mixture of primary care providers and private practice therapists deliver most of the mental health care to people with nonsevere mental disorders. For those with severe disorders, such as schizophrenia, bipolar disorder, and chronic depression, each of the 50 states oversees a public mental health program. Larger states often devolve responsibility to county or city authorities, so that there are actually multiple mental health care authorities and systems within many states. The only administrative commonality across states is funding by the federal Medicaid and Medicare programs for those who are impoverished, disabled, or aging. Medicaid is, however, administered differently in each state according to a variety of rules, regulations, and waivers. In addition to state public mental health programs, the federal government runs separate health care systems for active members of the military, for retired and disabled members of the military, and for Native Americans. For people with substance use disorders, the system is somewhat simpler, because the private sector is relatively small and the federal government supports most of the public care, with states contributing different amounts.

The organization of these many systems, programs, and providers is typically based on funding and profits rather than on public health needs, the preferences of users of the mental health services, or research. Few of the systems, programs, or individual practitioners collect data on quality or outcomes. Because so many providers, programs, and intermediaries (e.g. insurance agencies and managed care organizations) participate in the context of a largely private, for-profit system, health care costs are very large. The US health care system expenditures were approximately $2.5 trillion USD in 2009 [42]. Of this total, 5–12% has been devoted to behavioral health care in recent years [43]. The USA also spends much more than any other country on medical research. One advantage of the tremendous variation of programs and expenditures across regions has been the opportunity for innovation and research.

The community mental health movement began in the USA in 1963, when President John F. Kennedy signed the Community Mental Health Act and community mental health centers arose in towns and cities throughout the country [44]. Initially, these centers assumed too broad an agenda, including all mental health problems and prevention, as well as treatment. By the 1970s, community mental health programs narrowed their goals to treatment of persons with long-term and disabling illnesses, and facilitated deinstitutionalization of this population. Many long-term patients were transferred to group homes, nursing homes, and other institutions in the community, but the deinstitutionalization philosophy did result in significant downsizing of large state hospitals and of the total hospitalized population. The population in large public mental hospitals dropped from over 500 000 to less than 150 000 [44].

During the 1980s and 1990s, two movements strongly influenced community mental health care in the USA. The evidence-based practice movement arose from effectiveness research and evidence-based medicine, and, somewhat later, the recovery movement arose from the experiences of users of the mental health system.

The initial plan for community care, developed by the National Institute of Mental Health and termed the Community Support Program, centrally featured professional case managers, who would coordinate and broker all of the services for people with severe and persistent mental disorders in the community [45]. In the 1970s and 1980s, many challenges of caring for people in the community began to be apparent. Common concerns included integration and continuity of services for those with the most complex needs, appropriate housing, family burden, substance abuse and dependence, victimization, and violence [45]. More recently, unemployment, criminalization, and early mortality of people with mental illnesses have emerged as major concerns. All of these problems were exacerbated by poverty, reductions in housing subsidies, and shunting of people with mental illnesses into inner-city areas plagued by unemployment, crime, and drugs.

Many models of care were developed to address the special problems of people with SMDs living in the community [46]. For integration and continuity of care, assertive community treatment, intensive case management, clinical case management, and other models appeared. To address the need for housing, foster care, Fairweather Lodge, residential continuum, and supportive and supported housing models emerged. Likewise, other concerns were addressed by a variety of family interventions, treatments for cooccurring disorders, and so on. Research has supported some of these models and not supported others. Research-based models of care became identified as evidence-based practices. Various government reviews [47, 48] and systematic reviews [49–51] have identified specific interventions as evidence-based practices.

An additional concern has been the general failure to implement effective services in routine mental health treatment settings [52]. In 1997, the Robert Wood Johnson Foundation, the Substance Abuse and Mental Services Administration, several State Departments of Mental Health, and additional private foundations initiated a national demonstration to implement six specific evidence-based practices that were deemed essential community mental health services: systematic medication management, assertive community treatment, supported employment, family psych education, illness management and recovery, and integrated treatment for cooccurring disorders [53]. Because of research showing that faithfulness to evidence-based practices was strongly related to outcomes, the project emphasized implementation and fidelity. Outcomes showed that, with training and supervision for one year, most programs were able to implement and sustain high-quality evidence-based practices [54, 55]. Nevertheless, the degree of implementation of these practices varies widely from state to state [56].

The recovery movement, which typically encompasses opportunities for education, work, friendship, independent living, and community participation, has influenced numerous changes in community mental health care. Many states embrace recovery at the level of philosophy and mission, even if they have varying levels of success implementing its tenets. Rehabilitative services are more widely available, and many mental health programs have decreased the use of coercive measures, such as seclusion and restraint. The impact of the recovery movement has been much greater in some states than others [56].

In the 2000s, community mental health in the USA was dominated by attempts to control costs. These included managed care, fee-for-service systems, and Medicaid audits, which resulted in the government demanding that millions of dollars be returned. The financial recession severely affected state budgets and led to numerous cycles of financial cuts. The 15% of citizens without insurance (higher for those with mental illnesses) had great difficulty accessing even minimal care [57]. The net result has been a dramatic deterioration of community mental health care for people with the most severe disorders [47, 56, 58].

Very recently parity legislation and health care reform legislation have offered hope that people with mental illnesses in the USA will more easily acquire insurance, and that mental health disorders will be treated in the same manner as physical health disorders. How these two pieces of legislation are enacted over the next decade remains to be seen.

Canada

Analogously to the situation in the USA, each of Canada's ten provinces and three (northern) territories has its own mental health care system: health care for the great majority of the population falls under provincial and territorial jurisdiction. Nonetheless, several factors, including various institutional features common across all provinces, common proximity to the USA—which has had a major influence on service development in Canada [59, 60], federally managed equalization payments from richer to poorer provinces, and various mechanisms of exchange of information across provinces, have resulted in provincial mental health care systems bearing fairly close resemblance to one another. Partly due to equalization payments, perhaps partly also due to greater homogeneity in outlook concerning the resources needing to be allocated to the care of people with mental illness, per capita levels of funding for mental health are more similar across Canadian provinces than they are across the USA. Health care spending per capita in Canada is about half what it is in real terms in the USA. A recent report estimated that in 2003/4 total behavioral health spending in Canada was 5% of total health care spending, with per capita spending varying from $146 in Saskatchewan to $242 in New Brunswick and Alberta [61].

Common features of the Canadian mental health system include: (i) a mix of institutionally-based services delivered by unionized professionals and less regulated, nonunionized voluntary sector providers; (ii) universal coverage of hospital and physician services, as well as those of voluntary sector providers—but no public coverage of psychologists practicing independently; (iii) public coverage of medications for seniors and social assistance recipients, with some provinces providing varying levels of coverage for other people not covered by supplementary employer-based private insurance; (iv) physicians, including hospital-based psychiatrists, who are paid directly by provincial governments, mostly on a fee-for-service basis; (v) now with the notable exception of Alberta, regionalization of care delivery, resulting in further differentiation of community mental health services within individual provinces.

As in the USA, deinstitutionalization began in the late 1950s or early 1960s and was followed by the development of psychiatry departments within general hospitals. The voluntary sector quickly emerged to provide community-based care to the growing number of people with severe mental illness living in the community. Psychiatry departments and psychiatric hospitals gradually followed, adding community mental health services to their programming. This process has been slow, following the evidence-base with a lag measured in decades, and even today a number of psychiatry departments have hardly made a start. Access to evidence-based practices remains, as in the USA, rather limited.

There has been much discussion of recovery. Peer-support workers have become more commonly embedded into clinical services, and the notion that people with lived experience of mental illness should participate in administrative decisions and in research projects that have implications for them has gradually gained ground.

Some long-standing features of Canadian mental health care systems impede the development of high-quality community mental health care. Psychiatrists, who necessarily play a key role in community mental health care delivery, are paid directly by provincial governments independently of the quality of care they provide and have limited accountability. Union rules often seem designed to protect the privileges of members, especially those with more seniority, rather than serve the needs of clients. Funding for medications is open-ended, whilst funding for psychosocial services is severely constrained.

In 2006, after extensive consultation, the Standing Senate Committee on Social Affairs, Science and Technology tabled an influential report that painted a grim picture of the state of mental health and addiction services in Canada [62]. Services have not been well integrated and it is difficult, indeed often impossible, for people with mental illness and their caregivers to navigate successfully through them. Affordable, decent supportive or supported housing is often unavailable, as are integrated services for people with concurrent (mental illness and substance use) disorders, and employment services. Much more often than should be the case, what care is accessed is of questionable quality. Stigma is a common, disabling experience.

Following a key recommendation of the report, in 2007 the federal government established the Mental Health Commission of Canada, whose mandate is "to help bring into being an integrated mental health system that places people living with mental illness at its centre". Whatever its ultimate impact on provincial and territorial mental health policies and services, the Commission has stimulated an unprecedented sharing of ideas and perspectives across a broad range of stakeholders throughout the country.

Latin America and the Caribbean

Different models of mental health systems have been implemented in Latin American and Caribbean countries, though most of the initiatives have addressed a reduction in hospital beds and an increase of treatment within primary care. The Pan American Health Organization (PAHO) has started a cooperation initiative with those countries committed to the "Declaration of Caracas" (see Chapter 3)—the initiative for the restructuring of psychiatric care in Latin American and Caribbean countries—boosting the shift from hospital to community mental health care, through training human resources, providing research actions, and technical supervision [63]. Some progress in integrating mental health to community care has been observed mainly in Argentina, Brazil, Belize, Chile, Costa Rica, Cuba, El Salvador, Guatemala, Jamaica, Mexico, Nicaragua, and Panama [63–66].

A description of mental health systems and obstacles to their implementation within some countries of the region is given in Table 4.4. Some countries, such as Argentina, Belize, Cuba, and Jamaica, have invested in training of psychiatric nurses, guaranteeing mental health treatment in primary care services and making liaisons between community and mental health specialized services. Other countries, such as Brazil, Costa

Table 4.4 Summary of the favorable experiences and the main obstacles found in the implementation of community mental health services in a few Latin American and Caribbean countries.

LAC countries	Mental health systems	Obstacles
Argentina	• Almost half of the population is covered by the public sector, 47% by social security, and only 7.5% by the private sector. • Currently, there are 14 534 outpatient primary care services in the country, mostly financed by the public sector. • Rio Negro region: general doctors and nurses are the first to provide assistance for people with mental disorders and to refer them to a mental health team based in a general hospital. • Neuquén region: health workers and healers visit patients and families, and refer them to general doctors. In the Austral program, patients with mental disorders are seen by general doctors, and diagnosis is reached under psychiatric supervision.	• Psychiatrists have been resistant to shift from hospital to primary mental health care model [65]. • Conflicts and lack of cohesion among members of mental health teams [67]. • Irregular mental health supervision, lack of supervisors, and insufficient training to manage mental disorders [67]. • Shortage of specialized mental health professionals to refer patients [65]. • Budget has not been sufficient for basic needs such as telephone, fuel, and transportation, and there have been unstable supplies of medication [67]. • Lack of residential facilities for psychiatric patients discharged from hospitals [67]. • Transcultural barriers between outsider doctors and local beliefs and culture [65].
Belize	• Health system is compounded by 37 primary health centers, 3 polyclinics, 2 outpatient mental health services, 4 inpatient-psychiatric wards in general hospitals, and 8 general public hospitals. Also, there are 24-hour, 7-day emergency psychiatric services in all district hospitals. • People with mental health are assisted in primary care, mainly by psychiatric nurses under supervision of psychiatrists and psychologists [65, 128]. • Belize has introduced an outreach program, the Psychiatric Nurse Practitioner (PNP) in primary and secondary care, where nurses receive extensive training in mental health. • Psychiatric nurses are allowed to screen and to prescribe psychotropics under supervision and according to protocols and guidelines.	• Brain drain: nurses emigrate from Belize, seeking better working conditions in the UK and USA [128]. • Lack of budget for mental health and for basic needs (transportation for home visits) [65]. • Shortage of nurse visits [65]. • Burden on nurses (long working hours) [65].

(Continued)

Table 4.4 Continued.

LAC countries	Mental health systems	Obstacles
Brazil	• Mental health is integrated in the public health system through specialized teams in centers of psychosocial rehabilitation (CAPS), which are connected to family health programs in primary care and to psychiatric hospitals and psychiatric units in general hospitals [63, 69, 131]. • Primary health centers have general doctors trained to assist general mental health issues and, when necessary, to refer patients to specialized care such as CAPS or outpatient mental health care [131]. • Currently, almost 3000 long-stay inpatients who were discharged from psychiatric hospitals to sheltered homes receive public benefit payments (140 USD/month)—known as the "Return Home Program"—for their rehabilitation and social inclusion in the community [131]. • In Sobral, mental health care is provided by general doctors under supervision of mental health teams. • In Santos [68, 132] and Campinas [70, 71], CAPS are the main component of the systems and the majority of moderate and severe mental disorders are assisted in CAPS by specialized mental health teams.	• Low commitment to mental health issues by local government and health managers [129]. • Lack of or insufficient training and supervision in mental health [71, 130]. • Ideological conflicts among members of mental health teams and other health professionals [70]. • Stigma against people with mental disorders, especially related to renting houses for living and residential community services. • Lack of mental health professionals (psychiatrists) in emergency units during nights (CAPS) [71]. • Bureaucratic constraints to receiving benefits [129]. • Lack of national registers of people with mental disorders discharged from hospitals [130]. • CAPS and primary health care are not well integrated in many regions [130]. • Lack or insufficiency of residential facilities (sheltered homes) [129].
Chile	• The mental health system is based primarily in primary care and the use of general hospitals, though it includes psychiatric specialized teams and psychiatric hospitals. • Ambulatory mental health centers are often attached to general hospitals, and there are many group homes for deinstitutionalized and mentally ill persons across the country [74]. • Each service area is in charge of an assigned population within a geographical area [74].	• The Chilean Mental Health Society, a scientific organization for mental health professionals, has been opposed to the closure and transfer of beds [74]. • Resistance of mental health professionals to adherence to clinical guidelines [74]. • Insufficient computers and electronic databases to track the number of patients making use of services and having access to psychotropics [74].

Table 4.4 Continued.

LAC countries	Mental health systems	Obstacles
	• A mental health team comprises a psychiatrist, a psychologist, a social worker, an occupational therapist, a technical paramedic, and a health educator per 40 000 inhabitants. • Two programs of the National Mental Health Plan are directed to special populations: (i) treatment of depression nationwide; and (ii) comprehensive care for victims of the 17-year military dictatorship [133]. • Psychologists plus general practitioners follow the guidelines tested in a trial [73]; guidelines and treatment algorithms to treat depression across the country [74].	• The closure of beds has been viewed as a menace leading to loss of jobs by mental health professionals [74]. • Difficulties in referring severe cases of depression to specialized care; long waiting lists [74]. • Resources have been moved from the traditional preventive actions to the private sector, and a number of psychiatrists have moved to the private sector, which is now legally bound to cover this demand [134].
Cuba	• Havana city system: Covering an area of 46 000 people, one psychiatrist coordinates a mental health team that is integrated with family doctor care. • One of the greatest supports for the system is the participation and activity of popular associations. • The health system is based on family doctors spread out in the community, and operates at three levels of care: (i) community mental health centers, mental health teams in polyclinics, and the family doctor; (ii) psychiatric services in general hospitals where there are crisis intervention teams; and (iii) psychiatric hospitals.	• Lack of investment after US embargo and the decrease of participation of the USSR. • Low supply of medications.
Jamaica	• Health services are organized by regions, and general hospital wards are used to treat acute cases. General hospitals offer 24-hour emergency attendance. • Outpatient clinics are led by psychiatrists and Mental Health Officers (MHOs) [135].	• Difficulties contracting MHOs; the level of applicants is fairly high, and well-trained nurses are recruited to work in the USA [82]. • Some doctors are reluctant to send patients to MHOs [82]. • Violence in urban areas makes the work of MHOs more troublesome [82].

(Continued)

Table 4.4 Continued.

LAC countries	Mental health systems	Obstacles
	• An MHO is a specialized nurse practitioner who is trained in community psychiatry, psychology, social work, psychopharmacology, and patient management. • There are 41 MHOs in the country, and the average caseload is 500 patients. Nearly 200 patients can be seen by an MHO monthly [82].	• Lack of occupational therapists, insufficient assistance for housing, childcare, and rehabilitation [82]. • Two % of the mentally ill are homeless (60% of the homeless in the country) [82].
Mexico	• The system comprises Comprehensive Centers for Mental Health (CISAME), general health centers, shelters, and psychiatric units integrated in general hospitals.	• Resistance of health professionals to setting up of psychiatric wards in general hospitals [85]. • Insufficient residential facilities [85]. • Low budget for mental health care [85].

Rica, and Cuba, have invested in the training of general doctors in primary care under the supervision of mental health professionals. In Chile, mental health care is delivered for specific programs, such as care for depression and victims of violence, though public treatment is not offered to all citizens and for all mental disorders, leading to financial burdens on some patients and families.

Except for the smaller countries in the region, these models of care have been better implemented in regions with small populations, because they have attracted and trained more professionals providing community mental health care rather than referring patients to the big cities. The main obstacles in these regions have been financial constraints such as insufficient resources for the supply of medications, transport for home visits, adequate offices for care, as well as cultural resistance from both the community in accepting people with mental disorders and from health professionals in treating such patients (see Table 4.4). In the big cities, the implementation of community centers has been hindered mainly by political and ideological factors, inadequate infrastructures, a lack of integration amongst different levels of care, bureaucracy, legal constraints, and inefficient health and financial management.

Argentina

Psychiatric reform started in the 1980s, when the government set up health policies that focused on mental health, particularly in regards to long-stay hospital patients, and the development of therapeutic communities and psychiatric units in general hospitals. In 1983 there were 35 000 psychiatric beds in Argentina [67]; in 2008 this number had dropped to 16 000 [65]. Regional initiatives to close psychiatric hospitals begun in the 1990s were hindered following the financial crisis in 2003. Between 2004 and 2007 a Federal Health Plan was launched, giving priority to primary care. Each region in the country implemented its own mental health reform during this period, although overall the majority of regions kept a hospital-based care system.

Rio Negro and Neuquén in Patagonia are the main examples of regions where mental health has been integrated into community-based services [65, 67]. Rio Negro has 600 000 inhabitants, and changes in mental health services have advanced more there than in other regions of the country, especially after the approval of law 2440, in which treatment and rehabilitation were guaranteed for any person with a mental disorder. The only psychiatric public hospital (Neuropsiquiatrico de Allen) was closed in 1985, and a course in public mental health focusing on mental health services was developed to attract human resources in the region. Psychiatric beds were created in general hospitals, and halfway houses (residential services for long-stay patients who are discharged from psychiatric hospitals and do not have the option of living with family members) were opened [67].

Pathways of care include hospital-based emergency rooms, through referrals from primary doctors or nurses, with a mental health team being notified on call. Patients with mental disorders can be treated either at home or in general hospitals, community health centers, outpatient mental health offices, or halfway houses. The clearest benefit of Rio Negro's mental health program was the effect it had on policies, community institutions, and public attitudes towards mental disorders across the whole country.

Neuquén Province [65] has 350 000 inhabitants. Health reform in the region began in 1970, and since then the region has become the leading province in the promotion of community health care systems in Latin American and Caribbean countries. The province is divided into six zones, each with different levels of health care complexity. In rural areas, health workers visit patients and their families, and form links between them and the health system. Health workers and traditional healers are patients' first contact with the health system. General physicians are also an important component of the system, with specialists serving as consultants. Psychosocial rehabilitation is offered in most sites, and psychotherapy has been adapted according to the cultural context.

In 1995, the NGO-led AUSTRAL (Instituto Austral de Salud Mental rehabilitation program) program was launched. This program offered one-month to one-year training for several primary care physicians and other mental health professionals, beginning in 1996. Since 2000, more than 40 residents have been trained in general practice in Neuquén province. One consultant psychiatrist coordinates a journal club and provides mental health training and supervision by telephone. Moreover, the program offers community-based crisis intervention, rehabilitation, and maintenance of care, and also plays an important role in the reintegration of patients to society.

In the Neuquén region [65], approximately half of all primary general doctors use basic instruments to screen for depression and psychotic disorders. Thus, more people are being diagnosed and treated for these disorders. Between 1997 and 2006 the AUSTRAL program assisted 3200 people with mental health problems and their families. Overall, 12 000 people have benefitted from this program, and 80% of those in treatment in the AUSTRAL program have remained stable in the community. Only 5% of patients have required hospitalization since the AUSTRAL program has been implemented.

Overall, the main obstacles experienced in Argentina (see Table 4.4) are related to general doctors' resistance to treating mental disorders, ideological resistance from psychiatrists, insufficient supervision and training for general doctors and nurses, a tiny budget for basic needs, and an inadequate service infrastructure and low treatment coverage.

Belize

Belize is a lower middle-income country, located in Central America, with a population of 270 000 inhabitants. The only psychiatric hospital was closed in 2008 (Rockview Hospital), with technical support provided by PAHO. Nurses have been trained to provide mental health assistance in the community. They have been supervised by the only two psychiatrists available in the country, performing various tasks including assessment of patients, prescription of psychotropics, psychotherapy, consultation with local health and social agencies, consultation for teachers and school administrators, communication with families of clients, admitting and discharging of patients, assessing side-effects and efficacy of medications, working with staff to arrange activities for clients, and travelling to rural areas to provide care and home visits.

Mental health indicators (admissions/discharges, demographics, and diagnostic classification) have been integrated into the national Belize Health Information System in order to evaluate and monitor the provision of mental health services in the country. The success of the Belize system has in part been due to the efficiency in training psychiatric nurses in mental health care. The work conducted by the nurses [65] has been responsible for decreasing admissions to psychiatric hospitals, increasing outpatient-service consultations by 25%, and improving awareness of mental health issues in the health sectors and other sectors such as education and criminal justice.

The main obstacles to the implementation of mental health systems in Belize are related to brain drain, especially of psychiatric nurses, insufficiencies in the budget for basic needs, and burn-out among health professionals (see Table 4.4).

Brazil

Brazil is an upper middle-income country in South America, with a population of approximately 200 million. It is the leading economy in the region and the tenth largest economy in the world. The Unified Health System (Sistema Único de Saúde, SUS), created in 1988, includes as its principles universality, equity, and comprehensiveness. Public health systems are free of charge and available to all citizens in all Brazilian municipalities. Private health care is also available in the country, especially through health insurance, which is mainly sponsored by employers. However, only one-fifth of the population has access to private health insurance [65].

Brazilian psychiatric reform started in the 1990s, with the most remarkable changes being a 41% reduction of psychiatric beds between 1995 and 2005 [68,69] and an increase in the provision of community mental health services, though this is unequally distributed across the country [69]. In Brazil, the mental health system is based on offering mental health care through general medical doctors (Family Health Programme) within primary care, supervised by mental health teams placed in community psychosocial centers (CAPS).

The most successful cases of the integration of mental health into primary care in Brazil have occurred in two cities: Sobral and Campinas. Santos has also acted as a pioneer in closing an anachronic psychiatric hospital and in implementing community mental health care.

Sobral is a city with 175 000 inhabitants located in Ceara, a state in the north-east of Brazil. The economy is mainly based on commerce and agriculture, though industrial activities have been growing recently [65, 70]. There are two specialized community mental health centers (CAPS), one psychiatric emergency unit, one residential care facility (sheltered home), as well as primary health centers with Family Health Programmes. Patients with mental disorders are screened and treated by general doctors in family health teams, and only the most severe cases are referred to mental health specialists. These specialists provide mental health supervision to general doctors ("joint consultation") in how to manage patients with mental disorders. There is a strong connection between different levels of services. In Sobral the model of "joint consultation" has been successful in improving referral and management of mental disorders by general doctors.

Moreover, there has been a decrease in stigma against people with mental disorders and in resistance to offering assistance among general doctors, providing a better coverage of specialized community mental health care for people with moderate and severe mental disorders.

Campinas is a city in the state of Sao Paulo, in the south-east of Brazil, with a population of approximately one million. The process of deinstitutionalization started in 1990; since 1993, Candido Ferreira Hospital has served as a WHO mental health reference center. This hospital provides care for 1000 patients per month, and involves patients in income-generating projects and psychosocial rehabilitation programs [70]. Currently, the mental health system is compounded by six 24-hour specialized mental health community centers, with 32 psychiatric beds [71], and 30 mental health residential facilities, covering 150 patients discharged from long-stay psychiatric beds. Mental health teams provide support and technical supervision for health professionals in family health centers [72].

In Campinas, positive aspects of the specialized community mental health centers [71] have been described as follows: (i) patients were assisted by the same team during an acute crisis and in the follow-up phase of illness, which facilitated team–patient relationships and management; (ii) families were satisfied with specialized community mental health center services and home rescue; (iii) families were satisfied with group activities and considered them useful, informative, and supportive; and (iv) the reduction of beds was encouraging: from 1200 in 2003 to 250 in 2007 [70].

Santos is the biggest port in Latin America, situated in the state of Sao Paulo in the south-east of Brazil, with a population of approximately 420 000. Psychiatric reform started 20 years ago, after claims were made of torture and neglect of psychiatric patients in hospitals. Psychiatric hospitals were closed and community mental health services were implemented [68]. In 2005, the following actions helped foster mental health systems: (i) investments in developing community mental health units; (ii) an increase in the number of mental health workers; (iii) mental health training for health professionals; and (iv) the implementation of the national Return Home Programme, which covers benefits for long-stay patients discharged from psychiatric hospitals to residential services. In Santos the number of psychiatric hospitalizations has dramatically dropped, the coverage of community mental health care has substantially increased, and the supply of psychotropics is regular and available to all users [68].

Each region of the country has therefore adopted multiple models of community mental health care and its implementation has been heterogeneous, according to local political commitments, as well as financial and other resources. The obstacles in Brazil (see Table 4.4) include a variability of constraints for the implementation of services: stigma, ideological conflicts, lack of political commitment, lack of national registers of patients discharged from psychiatric hospitals, lack of human resources in some regions, and insufficient training in mental health.

Chile

The current population of Chile is around 16 million. The health care system is a public–private endeavor with a compulsory purchase of health insurance. Workers each decide whether to contribute to the public national health fund (FONASA, covering 68% of the population) or to one of over 20 private health insurers (Isapres). Chilean reform was triggered in 1993 when group homes were established for newly deinstitutionalized populations, and mental health programs were developed in day hospitals. In 1997 a mental health plan was developed by the Ministry of Health, based on priorities established through epidemiological studies, such as a clinical trial showing the efficacy of a stepped-care model to treat depression in primary care for low-income women [73], and a trial showing how depression can be treated on a large scale but at a low cost, leading to the transfer of knowledge from evidence to policy changes.

Psychologists have been incorporated into health teams in primary care, where mental health teams perform standardized diagnoses, promote education of patients and their families, use antidepressants in severe cases, deliver psychosocial sessions mainly to moderate and mild cases, and monitor and evaluate the feasibility and effectiveness of the program [74]. As a result of the implementation of these policies, 180 000 persons are beneficiaries of the victims program, over 60% of the estimated cases of depression have been receiving treatment, and the number of patients with access to antipsychotic medications has increased. Ideological conflicts and resistance from mental health professionals to the psychiatric reform have been the main constraints for the implementation of the new mental health care model.

Costa Rica

Costa Rica is located in Central America, with a population of around 4.6 million. It has been recognized for its leadership on health indexes, similar to those of developed countries. Health insurance (CCSS) in Costa Rica has universal coverage and incorporates mental health, including specific programs. The reform of health care in 1995 contributed effectively to increasing equity in access to primary care [75]. In 2007 the Ministry of Health implemented WHO-AIMS, which formed the basis for the evaluation and reformulation of mental health strategies [66]. The most important part of the mental health system is the primary care physicians' referral to one of the 135 psychiatrists in the country, who are located in 38 different facilities, including 26 psychiatric units in general hospitals, two psychiatric hospitals, and two day hospitals.

There are 812 sectors in the country with basic health teams (EBAIS—acronym in Spanish) comprising one general doctor, one nurse-auxiliary, one primary health care technician, one pharmacy technician, and one medical records technician. Evidence-based treatments are being incorporated into practice, primary care physicians are now better at identifying and treating individuals with depression, modern psychiatric medications are available to patients, and family members of patients have been organized into associations. However, many obstacles still have to be overcome: (i) there are still only a small number of mental health professionals in institutions for planning and decision-making [76]; (ii) Amerindian groups still require further attention, as there is inequity in community mental health services [77]; (iii) there is a scarcity of geriatric and child and adolescent psychiatrists [66]; and (iv) long-stay patients still remain in the National Psychiatric Hospital [78].

Cuba

Cuba has a population of around 11.4 million. The Caracas Declaration in 1990 (see Chapter 3) and the Havana Charter in 1995 both contributed to the reorientation of the mental health system, opening hospitals and giving the opportunity for patients to return home [79–81]. An important experience occurred in the Cienfuegos Province in 1996, after a hurricane destroyed a psychiatric hospital. Italian consultants participated in the reconstruction of the hospital, influencing the system to shift to a community- and individual-centered model. The empty wards were transformed into cultural centers opened to the community, or became sites for occupational therapies. Specialized units for acute admissions and emergencies were created for short-stay acute patients.

Community centers were designed to coordinate, organize, capacitate, and train human staff in mental health all across the country, which contributed to an increased coverage of the population (about 1 center to 30 000 people) [79]. The health system is based on family doctors spread out across the community, and operates at three levels of care: (i) the primary care level, comprising community mental health centers, mental health teams in polyclinics, and the family doctor; (ii) psychiatric services in general hospitals, where there are crisis intervention teams; and (iii) psychiatric hospitals [63].

Cuba has very strong communitarian organizations, with high levels of political access and influence. Cuba also has a long and deep tradition of community care centered on family doctors [63]. The mental health system is integrated and based on a general health system, with a solid communitarian constitution giving populations access and opportunities to participate in mental health care. Based on the communitarian pathway, the mental health system brings family and friends closer to patients. Psychiatric hospitals have been transformed to convivial places, and most people suffering from mental illness are now living in the community. The most important obstacle in this process has been the lack of investment after the US embargo and the subsequent economic crises, as the financial shortage made the provision of medicines and the hiring of mental health workers difficult.

Jamaica

The population of Jamaica is around 2.7 million. Its mental health system still centralizes many of its actions within large institutions, such as the Bellevue Hospital, a large hospital built in 1865 [82]. However, the population of Bellevue Hospital decreased by 58% between 1960 and 1990: from 3094 to 1296 patients [83]. Yearly admissions to Bellevue have been decreasing, and admission rates were reduced by 50% between 1971 and 1988. On the other hand, admissions to community mental health services increased from 7779 to 10 997 between 1995 and 2000 [82].

Specialized nurses assist patients in primary care and in outpatient clinics, led by psychiatrists and mental health officers (MHOs) [82]. The MHOs provide home treatment, assertive outreach and case management. They are not expected to initiate treatment but can reinstitute previous medicines in case of noncompliance. For those treated at home, medication is initiated in collaboration with a primary care doctor, and severe and more complex cases are referred to psychiatrists. When patients are admitted to hospital, the MHOs then visit them there, facilitating the liaison between the inpatient and the local psychiatrist. Referrals are made directly to the MHO or to a psychiatrist, though the majority of cases are initially seen by an MHO.

The main obstacles in Jamaica (see Table 4.4) are related to the resistance of medical doctors to referring patients to MHOs, and an insufficiency of services and human resources, causing burn-out of mental health professionals. Brain-drain of specialized nurses to the USA has also been a problem.

Mexico

The Mexican population is around 108 million. Although some asylums, such as La Castaneda, have been closed, the system is still generally centralized within hospitals. Only a very small proportion of those with a psychiatric diagnosis are being treated [84], probably as a result of the application of less than 1% of the total health budget to mental health [85].

The Hidalgo experience relates to the closure of the Ocaranza Asylum in 2000—an institution with a previous history of abuse and neglect of patients—located in Hidalgo State, a central region of Mexico with a population of 2.5 million. The strength of the program lies in the close connection to primary health care based on referral-counter systems, plus training and supervision for general health practitioners [85]. In 2000 there were 287 long-stay patients in the Ocaranza Asylum; after the hospital was closed 10 "villas" were built as residential alternatives, plus a 30-bed acute psychiatric ward and a 24-hour emergency ward. Although most patients were placed in the villas (34 were placed in halfway houses), 40% of the long-stay patients were transferred to other psychiatric hospitals. Prospective evaluation of long-stay patients discharged from the psychiatric hospitals shows that these patients have improved substantially in their daily living activities.

The main obstacles in Mexico have been the resistance of health professionals to include psychiatric beds in general hospitals, an insufficiency of services, and a lacking mental health budget (see Table 4.4).

South Asia

Across the South Asia region, for centuries the mentally ill were managed by the community in several ways, ranging from physical restraint through use of chains to ancient medical treatment systems such as Ayurveda. Asylums or mental hospitals were introduced under British rule in India and through the colonization of other South Asian countries. Although they provided some treatment and relief for the mentally ill, they were also edifices of neglect, abuse, and human rights violations. Whilst many such hospitals in South Asia have undergone changes for the better, some of them still retain the old character and are largely custodial in their function. In India, the 42 mental hospitals cater to a mere 20% of the population, all in urban areas [86], with no services available for the other, predominantly rural, 80%.

The centralization of the mental health delivery system has received a major setback in recent years and the focus has now shifted to community care rather than creating new mental asylums. Many reasons have been identified for the failure of mental asylums in the South Asian region, including ill-treatment of patients, geographical and professional isolation, poor reporting and accounting, bad management, poorly targeted financial resources, lack of staff training, and inadequate quality assurance procedures.

It is only in the last 30–40 years that some attempts have been made to establish community-based care in many countries of the region. In India, general hospital psychiatry units were set up in the 1960s, followed by the drafting of the National Mental Health Program (NMHP) in 1982 (see Chapter 5 for details). The program envisaged deinstitutionalization and the integration of mental health care with primary care [87]. The WHO's technical report in 1990 [88] also provided an impetus for community-care programs. A series of other initiatives, such as initiation of community or satellite clinics, domiciliary care programs, and the training of school teachers, volunteers, and village leaders in early identification of mental disorders, also helped galvanize the community programs. Family wards, where family members can stay with admitted patients and take part in the treatment process, have been another step in this direction, although they have been initiated only in a few teaching centers. NGOs have also played a role in the growth of community care. Some have their own community-based programs and cater to a variety of conditions [89]. It is a pity that they work in isolation and their resources are not being utilized by the governments for private–public partnerships.

The concept of community care has brought into focus individual-based care and treatment, a wider range of services, coordinated treatment programs, services closer to home, ambulatory care, and partnership with caregivers. However, several studies in the region have highlighted the large number of untreated patients in the community. Even the existing services are under-utilized, due to varied explanatory models held by patients and their families [90], which result in them seeking help from religious and traditional healing sites.

Mental health issues may be tackled and delivery may be improved through better cooperation among the regional countries. Partnership is needed in areas such as research, organizing community care, health education, public awareness through media, publication of data, training programs, exchanges of faculty/postgraduate trainees, integration with general health care, training primary care physicians, national mental health programs, teaching psychiatry to undergraduate medical students, general hospital psychiatry, and enlisting the cooperation of the private sector/NGOs.

Bangladesh

Mental health is part of the primary health care system. Treatment of SMDs is available at the primary level, and efforts are being made to provide cheaper drugs at the primary level. Regular training of primary care professionals is being carried out in the field of mental health. Mental health training for primary care physicians and health workers is being conducted by the Ministry of Health and Family Welfare; they are trained to develop biological, psychological, and social orientation towards all health problems, diagnostic skills, skills in data collection, and the ability to train other mental health staff in turn.

There are community care facilities for patients with mental disorders. Periodic mental health extension services are being provided at the primary care level by the Institute of Mental Health Research, Dhaka. Public education and family counseling are conducted with the supervision of specialists. Though specific rehabilitation programs are not available in an organized form, efforts are being made to implement day-care facilities, sheltered workshops, and rehabilitation programs for people with chronic schizophrenia [91].

The Bangladeshi Mental Health Association is an NGO involved in mental health care in Bangladesh [92]. This NGO aims to promote and provide a culturally appropriate community-based mental health service to the people of Bangladesh, to counter all kinds of violence, encourage self-support through mental health education and education in consequences, and to promote social inclusion.

Bhutan

Under the surmise that, with the existence of a fairly well developed primary health care system, a community-based mental health care system was likely to succeed, various strategies were adopted, including an integration of mental health care services into existing general care services. The first priority was to identify specific activities to be carried out at different levels of health care facilities, such as hospitals and basic health units. Accordingly, training programs for different levels of health workers were developed and implemented. At the same time, advocacy and public awareness programs were launched to sensitize government leaders and the public.

Essential psychotropic drugs were included in the essential drugs program and supplied to health facilities. Several batches of district medical officers have provided basic psychiatric skills training; they now provide basic psychiatric services in the district hospitals. Many nurses have participated in the training and orientation course on mental health. The essential drugs list was revised to include psychiatric drugs at the level of district hospitals and basic health units. Entries on CMDs have been included in the Standard Treatment Manual for health workers. CMDs are included in the general health information reporting system. Lastly, collaborative work on mental health issues has commenced with the education, welfare, and law enforcement sectors.

At the community level, among other activities, a pilot study on community knowledge, attitudes, and practices concerning mental health was conducted. Representatives from traditional healers ("Drungtshos") and religious leaders were included in the survey—in planning, focus-group discussions, and the field survey. This experience of modern and traditional health practitioners working together gave important additional understanding of each other's perspectives on mental health, and of how to work more closely together in the future. The survey also proved to be valuable hands-on training for the health workers, who hitherto did not have much experience in detecting mental disorders. The survey process likewise sensitized the community to mental illnesses. Therefore, it was a learning experience for both surveyors and community representatives. This method of consultation with community leaders also indicated that they could be trained to identify mental disorders in the community. Because of the survey, many new patients are receiving treatment, underscoring the links with gross national happiness (GNH) [93]. Numerous challenges remain for mental health needs, requiring further positive steps in development.

India

Non-institutional care, a core concept of community psychiatry, has always been practiced in India through the ages, although it has been rather disorganized in structure and in function [94]. Essentially, most community-based mental health care in the country has been a biomedical psychiatric service approach. However, community-based rehabilitation, envisaged as an important component of the community mental health care system, needs to be sensitive to social and cultural influences. Emphasis should lie on the adoption of simple psychosocial strategies rather than structured technical approaches. The scope of vocational rehabilitation is enormous in the large agro-rural community in India. The onus of initiating CBR programs for the mentally ill has largely rested on NGOs [95].

A strong commitment to extending care into the community has resulted in the active involvement of NGOs in community outreach [96]. Several community mental health programs have been reported in various parts of the country [97–99]. These programs, operated by voluntary agencies and NGOs, have been demonstrated to be feasible and cost-effective [97, 100]. Although NGOs have a substantial amount of commitment and drive, the continued sustenance of these programs is dependent on funding, which is often timebound. Many NGOs are either not interested in, or cannot afford an external evaluation of their programs.

Maldives

Mental health is not part of a primary health care system, and treatment of SMDs is not available at the primary level. Regular training of primary care professionals is carried out in the field of mental health; the WHO has developed a video-based teaching module for mental health which can be used as a learning tool by doctors even in outlying islands. Training in mental health is also integrated into the community health workers' training program.

Specialized mental health care is available only in the capital, Male. Each island has a medical center staffed by an expatriate doctor. At the atoll and island levels, trained community health workers and nurses provide basic psychiatric care and home-based care for patients, and promote mental health through awareness-raising.

There are six NGOs actively involved in mental health-related work, including the rehabilitation of children with learning disabilities, awareness programs for parents with mentally and physically disabled children, outreach programs for substance abusers, the teaching of life skills to students, programs for the well-being of the elderly, provision of psychosocial support, and resilience-building around social issues.

Nepal

In Nepal religious and traditional beliefs determine help-seeking behaviors. The stigma of mental illness drives people to religious rather than psychiatric help. Families bear the brunt of care, and funding for mental health services is grossly inadequate. Mental health training has been provided to general health professionals by the WHO regional office [101].

One NGO is running a community mental health service in 7 of the 75 districts in the country. In these districts, primary health care workers have received mental health training and refresher trainings. In other districts, community mental health services are not available, as mental health care is not yet integrated into the general health service system.

The Centre for Mental Health and Counselling—Nepal (CMC-Nepal) is a national-level NGO, registered on 1 May 2003 in the Kathmandu District Administration Office and affiliated to the Social Development Council. It is working on various levels with preventive, promotive, and curative aspects of mental health, aiming to provide mental health services in the community. It is also supporting other organizations in their psychosocial programs. The initiator of CMC-Nepal is United Mission to Nepal, Mental Health Program, established in 1984.

The community mental health and psychosocial support program aims to make mental health services available as an integrated part of the existing health system and promotes mental health issues in 17 districts. NGOs are supported in addressing the psychosocial needs of traumatized people in their program areas. Program activities include:

- Basic and refresher training in mental health for doctors and paramedic staff, with supervision visits and meetings.
- Training in basic listening skills, trauma-related issues, and counseling for local NGO staff, with regular supervision.
- Awareness-raising activities (radio programs, exhibitions, and health camps).
- Seed money for psychotropic drugs.
- A charity fund for poor chronic epileptic and psychotic patients.

The Child Mental Health Programme promotes mental health among children and adolescents in Dolakha and Kavre districts, and facilitates the provision of mental health services for those with emotional and behavioral problems. The aim is to integrate this approach within the government district education and health systems. Program activities include:

- Training and supervision of teachers, student volunteers, and supervisors in preventative and promotive approaches for the psychosocial well-being of children and adolescents.
- Support for reading and play materials.
- Life-skills education for children and adolescents.
- Training and supervision of health workers in child and adult mental health.
- A Child Guidance Clinic in the Charikot Primary Health Care Centre, Dolakha.

Pakistan

The situation in Pakistan is somewhat similar to that in Nepal. Religious healers, hakims, and homeopaths have a role to play in the management of mental disorders. The clinic-based primary health care system does not allow for a formal referral pattern. A rural community-based mental health program has been one recent initiative: it includes data collection, training, development of referral systems, and evaluation of outcome [102].

There are 3729 outpatient mental health facilities in the country, of which 1% are for children and adolescents only. These facilities treat 343.34 users per 100 000 general population. The average number of contacts per user is 9.31. Of these outpatient facilities, 46% provide follow-up care in the community, whilst 1% have mental health mobile teams. In terms of available interventions, 1–20% of users have received one or more psychosocial interventions in the past year.

Many (624) community-based psychiatric inpatient units are available in the country, for a total of 1.9 beds per 100 000 population. Very few (1%) of these beds in community-based inpatient units are reserved for children and adolescents only [103]. 75% of admissions to community-based psychiatric inpatient units are female and 18% are children/adolescents. The diagnoses of admissions to community-based psychiatric inpatient units were primarily from the following two diagnostic groups: mood (affective) disorders (46%), and neurotic, stress-related and somatoform disorders (32%). On average, patients spend 17 days per discharge. Some 1–20% of patients in community-based psychiatric inpatient units received one or more psychosocial interventions in the last year. A total of 34% of community-based psychiatric inpatient units had at least one psychotropic medicine of each therapeutic class (antipsychotic, antidepressant, mood-stabilizer, anxiolytic, and antiepileptic medicines) available in the facility. Community residential facilities are not available in the country.

Over the last 17 years Pakistan has developed a community-based program of mental health care delivery in a phased manner, aimed at providing a balanced model of care for countries with limited resources and faced with the double burden of communicable and noncommunicable illnesses. During the first phase, a preliminary evaluation was made of the needs and demands for mental health services in the community, to gauge the knowledge, attitude, and practices of the community, and to educate them by using mosques, social congregations, and faith healers. This was followed by the reparation of training and teaching materials for primary health care personnel and education materials for the community. The next phase involved oral collaborations for the promotion of mental health and the prevention of mental illnesses. Education administrators were sensitized to the need to incorporate mental health principles in order to improve the quality of education. This activity has now been completed at the national level. The next stage involves the development of a training package for schoolteachers, which has been carried out in a decentralized manner. The response of school teachers and children is overwhelming, with the formation of the All Pakistan Teachers' Movement for mental health being one success. Faith healers have also been provided with colored case-identification cards, similar to those used by multipurpose health workers, and they act as an important source of referral to health care facilities.

Sri Lanka

In Sri Lanka, community mental health programs were activated and expanded after the tsunami in 2005. They have also been linked with primary care services, with a focus on education and prevention. The WHO initiated community-based rehabilitation projects in three areas and an evaluation has been completed [104].

More than three decades of conflict and the effects of the tsunami are having a strong impact on the mental well-being of the Sri Lankan population, especially in its most deprived sectors. Mental health data from Sri Lanka shows an increase in SMDs and CMDs in times of armed conflict. This country has one of the highest suicide rates in the world. Further, misuse of alcohol is frequent, especially in areas affected by disaster. It is estimated that 3% of the Sri Lankan population suffer from some kind of mental disorder. At the same time, mental health services have hardly developed in conflict-affected and other areas. Thus, access to mental health services is extremely limited and grossly disproportionate from one area of the country to another. Mental health care is still mainly concentrated and provided in large psychiatric hospitals in Colombo and the areas surrounding it. Very frequently, big psychiatric institutions have been a major issue for human rights concerns. In spite of this grave situation, insufficient attention is given to the mental health sector, and at times it is entirely forgotten. Improving people's mental health and psychosocial well-being is one of the priority objectives of WHO Sri Lanka's 2006–2011 Country Strategy. Therefore, the WHO is working closely with the Ministry of Healthcare and Nutrition on the development of a mental health assistance program that may provide special attention to the most underserved sectors of the population. A survey of 152 LAMICs showed that only three countries in the world—namely Sri Lanka, Chile, and Brazil—have shown a national level of success with mental health interventions.

East and South-East Asia

Balance of hospital/community care

As balance indicator of hospital and community care in the region, the number of psychiatrists and psychiatric beds per 10 000 people is displayed in Figure 4.1 (except for East Timor). This ratio is commonly used as an indicator of hospital care, whilst the number of psychiatrists per population represents potential community care. Interestingly, there is a significant positive correlation between the number of psychiatrists and number of beds in the region (Pearson correlation coefficients $= 0.95$, $p < 0.001$).

Japan had the highest number of psychiatrists per 10 000 people in the region (9.4) at the time of the WHO report in 2005 [2], followed by South Korea (3.5), Mongolia (3.3), and Singapore (2.3). Despite a decrease in recently admitted patients, Japan (28.4) also has significantly more beds than other countries in the region, followed by South Korea (13.8). Mongolia is another country which maintains a hospital-based care system, with an occupancy rate of above 80% [105].

Community care at the primary care level

In low-resource countries, delivery of mental health care is focused on the primary care level. Essential elements of this stage comprise: (i) screening and assessment by primary care staff; (ii) talking treatments, including counseling and advice; (iii) pharmacological treatment; (iv) liaison with and training by mental health specialist staff, where available; and (v) limited specialist back-up available for training, consultation for complex cases, and inpatient assessment and treatment for cases that cannot be managed in primary care [24, 31].

Nongovernmental organizations

NGOs assist the least-resourced countries in the region in providing mental health care. International NGOs have set up model mental health services, and trained both health care and non-health workers in post-conflict countries such as Cambodia and East Timor, where all mental health

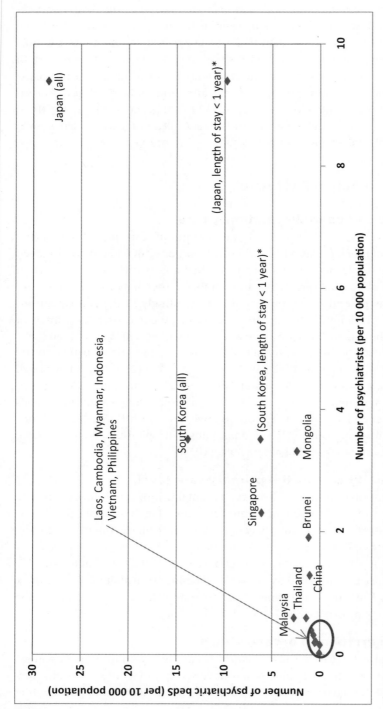

Figure 4.1 Number of psychiatrists and psychiatric beds in the East and South-East Asia region.
*Number of psychiatric beds for patients who stayed less than 1 year in South Korea and Japan.
Data from [2, 136–138].

resources were destroyed [2, 106, 107]. In Malaysia, local NGOs provide residential care, day-care services, and psychosocial rehabilitation services in the community [105]. In the Philippines, collaborative activities between local NGOs and university groups compensate for the government's limitations [108]. Most NGOs' activities cover (i) screening and assessment and (ii) talking treatments. Psychological—rather than Western-style pharmacological—treatment is popular in these countries.

Mental health within public health

Mental health services are often integrated into the public health system across the region. In Malaysia and Thailand, community mental health promotion and prevention activities are conducted through public places, such as schools, churches, temples, and community halls [105]. In countries such as Japan, Singapore, and South Korea, health centers provide psychological counseling, screening for mental health problems, and psychoeducation, whilst day centers offer vocational rehabilitation and mental health promotion activities by multidisciplinary teams.

Asia is vulnerable to natural disasters, including earthquakes and floods. Although the deadliest earthquakes hit this area, these tragic disasters have also deepened awareness of the need to develop community mental health systems. Mental health and psychosocial support are included in disaster preparedness in Indonesia [109], Myanmar [110], and Thailand [111]. Such aid has led to the development of a national guideline for mental health interventions in disasters [111], and a community mental health nursing (CMHN) training program [112].

General mental health care level

Medium-resource countries in the region have generally established a range of service components. At the general mental health care level, these may include: (i) outpatient/ambulatory clinics; (ii) community mental health teams; (iii) acute inpatient care; (iv) long-term community-based residential care; and (v) employment and occupation support (see Appendix A for details). In addition, case management is necessary amongst case managers, primary physicians, and mental health specialists [24, 31].

Outpatient/ambulatory clinics are increasing in many countries, especially those with greater numbers of psychiatrists, such as Japan, South Korea, and Singapore. Community-based mental health teams provide outreach services for large populations outside of hospitals, including visiting nursing programs and case management. Acute care is available in medium- or high-resource countries, though the coordination between hospital and community services, such as the provision of referral systems, is weak. Many countries provide long-term community-based residential care; this is available in all countries except Indonesia, Laos, the

Philippines, and Thailand [2]. Chronic beds for long-stay patients are being converted into residential facilities and group homes in communities, such as private nursing homes in Malaysia [113]. Employment support programs to find and retain work are provided at day-care centers and assist persons with depression return to work [114].

Specialized mental health care

In medium- or high-resource countries, specialized clinics are available for specific disorders, including eating disorders, dual diagnosis, and substance abuse, and adolescent problems in medium- or high-resource countries. In Singapore, the National Addictions Management Service (NAMS) provides care for patients with addiction disorders in the community through a multidisciplinary team [115].

Home-care and day-hospital services are used as alternatives to hospital admission. In Singapore, a mobile crisis team (community nurses assisted by a medical officer or a medical social worker) conducts home visits for crisis intervention, whilst community psychiatric nursing teams offer home care to discharged patients living in the community, including assessment and monitoring, as well as psychological support for caregivers [116].

In China, psychiatric hospitals send professionals to the homes of people with SMDs to provide "home-bed" services [117, 118]. For people with chronic mental disorders, sheltered workshops for their rehabilitation and "rural guardianship network" for their supervision and management are also available, though the effectiveness of these alternative services is controversial [118, 119]. In China, nongovernment services such as private psychiatric clinics, nonprofessional counseling clinics, telephone hotlines, and folk treatments are becoming the dominant form of community mental health service, although their sustainability is of concern [120].

Most early intervention and assertive community treatments are provided in pilot specialized community mental health projects. In the Philippines, more than 7000 patients were hospitalized in the National Mental Hospital in Manila; however, the introduction of acute crisis intervention services (ACIS) reduced this number by more than half [121].

Assertive community treatment (ACT) provides assertive and comprehensive community-based services by a multidisciplinary team to people with severe and persistent mental disorders (see Appendix A for details). Japan, South Korea, Singapore, and Malaysia have introduced ACT with cultural modifications. ACT models are usually assessed with key outcome measures, such as length of stay, hospital readmission rate, and quality of life. A Japanese study in pre- and post-pilot phase reported a reduction in length of stay, whilst a subsequent randomized clinical trial showed a decrease in inpatient days and higher CSQ-8 scores in an ACT group compared to a control group [122]. In South Korea, ACT staff members play roles as both care managers of ACT and health workers in community mental health centers. In a pre–post comparison, the number and duration of admissions were also dramatically reduced, and the clinical and social outcomes were significantly improved [123, 124]. In Singapore, the ACT program was effective in reducing the frequency and duration of admissions in a clinical trial. The employment status of patients also showed improvement over the course of study [125].

Key points in this chapter

- In the Africa region, generally specialized psychiatric hospitals are the mainstay of treatment for the mentally ill, with only around half of the countries in the region reporting having community-based mental health care. Whilst there has been a move towards the decentralization of specialist mental health services in some countries, the level of integration of mental health is usually limited. Whilst the majority of countries in the region claim to have mental health care integrated into primary health care services, evidence for this actually being the case is limited, though there is substantial heterogeneity across countries.
- In Australia and New Zealand, there is a comprehensive mix of hospital and community-based services available overall, though there is variability in the access patients may have to such services within both countries (in particular Australia, for instance according to location). In the Pacific Island Nations, mental health services are significantly underdeveloped, with services being delivered mainly through village- or community-based primary health care clinics, linked in some cases to regional clinics or national hospitals. However, there has been some progress in recent years through PIMHnet.
- In the European region, there has been an overall trend towards an increase in community-based mental health services and a decrease in institutional care. However, the pace and scale at which this is occurring, as well as the quality of services, varies widely. Whilst in the high-income (mostly Western) countries a large array of multidisciplinary community-based services may be available, with most patients being treated outside of mental institutions, in the low-income or lower middle-income (Eastern) countries mental health institutions are commonly still the mainstay of the mental health care system. Although some mental health care is available in primary care settings in all countries of the region, these services are often inadequate.
- In the USA, most of the mental health treatment for nonsevere mental disorders is provided through a mixture of primary care providers and private practice therapists, and for severe disorders is provided through

regional public mental health programs. The organization of these many systems, programs, and providers is typically based on funding and profits. In Canada, health care also mostly falls under provincial and territorial jurisdiction.

- In Latin American and Caribbean countries, there has been a general reduction in hospital beds and an increase of treatment within primary care, though various models of mental health systems have been implemented across different countries. The main obstacles in the region to the implementation of mental health care have been financial constraints, cultural resistances, political and ideological factors, inadequate infrastructures, a lack of integration amongst different levels of care, bureaucracy, legal constraints, and inefficient health and financial management.

- In the South Asia region, the focus in most countries has now shifted to community care rather than the creation of new mental asylums. However, whilst many of the hospitals that still exist have undergone changes for the better, some of them are still severely inadequate and largely custodial in their function. Furthermore, there is a large number of untreated patients in the community across the region. NGOs play a significant role in the implementation of community mental health services, though they often work in isolation.

- In the East and South-East Asia region, there is large variability across countries in community mental health services available. In low-resource countries, delivery of mental health care is primarily focused on the primary care level, with NGOs providing further services. Medium-resource countries generally have a range of service components available, including increasingly outpatient/ambulatory clinics. In medium- or high-resource countries, specialized clinics are also available for specific disorders, as well as home care, day-hospital services, early intervention and assertive community treatments, and ACT.

References

[1] Institute of Medicine. Mental, Neurological, and Substance Use Disorders in Sub-Saharan Africa: Reducing the Treatment Gap, Increasing Quality of Care—Workshop Summary. Washington DC: Institute of Medicine; 2010.

[2] World Health Organization. Mental Health Atlas, revised edition; 2005.

[3] World Health Organization and Wonca. Integrating mental health into primary care—A global perspective. Geneva: WHO and World Organization of Family Doctors; 2008.

[4] Kgosidintsi, A. The role of the community mental health nurse in Botswana: the needs and problems of carers of schizophrenic clients in the community. Curationis 1996;19(2):38–42.

[5] Moosa MYH, Jeenah FY. Community psychiatry: An audit of the services in southern Gauteng. South African Journal of Psychiatry 2008;14(2):36–43.

[6] Petersen I. Comprehensive integrated primary mental health care for South Africa: Pipedream or possibility? Social Science & Medicine 2000;51(3):321–34.

[7] Stein DJ, Allwood C, Emsley RA. Community care of psychiatric disorders in South Africa: Lessons from research on deinstitutionalisation. South African Medical Journal 1999;89(9):942–3.

[8] Freeman M, Lee T, Vivian W. Evaluation of mental health services in the Free State—Part III: Social outcome and patient perceptions. South African Medical Journal 1999;89(3):311–15.

[9] Freeman M, Lee T, Vivian W. Evaluation of mental health services in the Free State—Part IV: Family burden and perspectives. South African Medical Journal 1999;89(3):316–18.

[10] Kilonzo GP, Simmons N. Development of mental health services in Tanzania: A reappraisal for the future. Social Science & Medicine 1998;47(4):419–28.

[11] Erinosho OA. Mental health delivery-systems and post-treatment performance in Nigeria. Acta Psychiatrica Scandinavica 1977;55(1):1–9.

[12] Cohen, A. The effectiveness of mental health services in primary care: the view from the developing world. Geneva: WHO; 2001.

[13] Agomoh AO, Onwukwe JU, Acho, Eaton J. Scaling-up a successful community mental health programme in South-East Nigeria. World Psychiatric Association Regional Meeting: "Scaling up and reaching down—addressing unmet need for services". Abuja, Nigeria: African Association of Psychiatrists and Allied Professions; 2009.

[14] BasicNeeds. Community mental health practice: Seven essential features for scaling up in low- and middle-income countries. Bangalore; 2009.

[15] Petersen I, Pillay YG. Facilitating community mental health care in South Africa—the role of community health workers in the referral system. South African Medical Journal 1997;87(11):1621–6.

[16] Thom R. Mental health services research review final report (Grant 256/00). South Africa: Health Systems Trust; 2003.

[17] Meissner O. The traditional healer as part of the primary health care team? South African Medical Journal 2004;94(11):901–2.

[18] Robertson BA. Does the evidence support collaboration between psychiatry and traditional healers? Findings from three South African studies. South African Psychiatry Review 2006;9:87–90.

[19] Adiibokah E, Doku V, Eaton J. Factors associated with successful establishment of independent Mental Health Self-Help Groups in West Africa—WPA Psychiatric Association Regional Meeting: "Scaling up and reaching down—addressing unmet need for services". Abuja, Nigeria: African Association of Psychiatrists and Allied Professions; 2009.

[20] Makhale MS, Uys LR. An analysis of support groups for the mentally ill as a psychiatric intervention strategy in South Africa. Curationis 1997;20(1):44–9.

[21] Department of Health and Aging. National Mental Health Report: Summary of 15 years of reform Canberra. Commonwealth of Australia; 2010.

[22] Mental Health Commission. Blueprint for Mental Health Services in New Zealand. New Zealand: Mental Health Commission; 1998.

[23] Mental Health Council of Australia. Not For Service: Experiences of Injustice and Despair in Mental Health Care in Australia. Canberra: Mental Health Council of Australia; 2005.

[24] Thornicroft G, Tansella M. Components of a modern mental health service: A pragmatic balance of community and hospital care—Overview of systematic evidence. British Journal of Psychiatry 2004;185:283–90.

[25] Hughes F. Report to the World Health Organisation on Developing a Technical Support Programme for the Organisation of Mental Health Services in the Western Pacific Region. Mary Finlayson. Auckland, New Zealand: Centre for Mental Health Research, Policy and Service Development. Patrick Firkin; 2005.

[26] Desjarlais R, Eisenberg L, Good B, Kleinman A. World Mental Health: Problems and Priorities in Low-Income Countries; New York: Oxford University Press; 1995.

[27] Heywood DA. Review of New Zealand's Development Assistance to the World Health Organization (WHO) Pacific Islands Mental Health Network (PIMHnet)2005–2008, NZAID. NZAID Evaluation & Research Report Collection. World Health Organisation; 2009.

[28] Rosen A. Is the IVth Mental Health Plan a dud? Croakey: the Crikey Health Site; 2009.

[29] Thornicroft G, Tansella M. Balancing community-based and hospital-based mental health care. World Psychiatry 2002;1:84–90.

[30] Thornicroft G, Tansella M. What are the arguments for community-based mental health care? Copenhagen: WHO Regional Office for Europe; 2003.

[31] Thornicroft G, Tansella M. Better Mental Health Care. Cambridge: Cambridge University Press; 2009.

[32] Thornicroft G, Tansella M, Law A. Steps, challenges and lessons in developing community mental health care. World Psychiatry 2008;7:87–92.

[33] World Health Organization. Policies and Practices for Mental Health in Europe: Meeting the Challenges. WHO; 2008.

[34] Knapp M, McDaid D, Mossialos E, Thornicroft G. Mental Health Policy and Practice Across Europe: An Overview. In: Knapp M, McDaid D, Mossialos E, Thornicroft G, editors. Mental Health Policy and Practice Across Europe. Maidenhead: Open University Press; 2007. pp. 1–14.

[35] European Commission. The State of Mental Health in the European Union. European Commission; 2004.

[36] World Health Organization. Mental Health: Facing the Challenges, Building Solutions—Report from the WHO European Ministerial Conference. Copenhagen: WHO Regional Office for Europe; 2005.

[37] World Health Organization. WHO-AIMS Report on Mental Health System in Armenia. Yerevan, Armenia: WHO and Ministry of Health; 2009.

[38] NHS Centre for Reviews and Dissemination. Effective Health Care: Improving the Recognition and Management of Depression in Primary Care (Rep. No. 7 (5)). 2002.

[39] World Health Organization. WHO-AIMS Report on Mental Health System in the Kyrgyz Republic. Bishkek, Kyrgyz Republic: WHO and Ministry of Health; 2008.

[40] World Health Organization. Mental Health Services in Europe: The Treatment Gap Briefing Paper, WHO European Ministerial Conference on Mental Health, Helsinki, 12–15 January 2005.

[41] World Health Organization. Mental Health Gap Action Programme: Scaling Up Care for Mental, Neurological, and Substance Use Disorders; 2008.

[42] Centers for Medicare and Medicaid Services. National health care expenditures data. Baltimore: Centers for Medicare and Medicaid Services; 2010.

[43] Frank R, Goldman H, McGuire T. Trends in mental health cost growth: an expanded role for management? Health Affairs 2009;28:649–59.

[44] Dixon L, Goldman H. Forty years of progress in community mental health: the role of evidence-based practices. Australian and New Zealand Journal of Psychiatry, 2003;37:668–73.

[45] Turner J, TenHoor W. The NIMH community support program: pilot approach to a needed social reform. Schizophrenia Bulletin, 1978;4:319–48.

[46] Corrigan P, Mueser K, Bond G, Drake R, Solomon P. The principles and practice of psychiatric rehabilitation. New York: Guilford; 2008.

[47] New Freedom Commission on Mental Health. Achieving the promise: transforming mental health care in America. Rockville: US Department of Health and Human Services; 2003.

[48] US Department of Health and Human Services. Mental health: a report of the Surgeon General. Rockville: US Department of Health and Human Services; 1999.

[49] Chambless D, Ollendick T. Empirically supported psychological interventions: controversies and evidence. Annual Review of Psychology 2001;52:685–716.

[50] Cook J. Blazing new trails: using evidence-based practice and stakeholder consensus to enhance psychosocial rehabilitation services in Texas. Psychiatric Rehabilitation Journal 2004;27:305–6.

[51] Kreyenbuhl J, Buchanan RW, Dickerson FB, Dixon LB, Schizophrenia Patient Outcomes Research Team (PORT). The Schizophrenia Patient Outcomes Research Team (PORT): updated treatment recommendations 2009. Schizophrenia Bulletin 2010;36:94–103.

[52] Torrey W, Drake R, Dixon L, Burns BJ, Flynn L, Rush AJ, et al. Implementing evidence-based practices for persons with severe mental illnesses. Psychiatric Services 2001;52:45–50.

[53] Drake R, Goldman H, Leff H, Lehman AF, Dixon L, Mueser KT, et al. Implementing evidence-based practices in routine mental health service settings. Psychiatric Services 2001;52:179–82.

[54] McHugo G, Drake R, Whitley R, Bond GR, Campbell K, Rapp CA, et al. Fidelity outcomes in the national implementing evidence-based practices project. Psychiatric Services 2007;58:1279–84.

[55] Swain K, Whitley R, McHugo G, Drake R. The sustainability of evidence-based practices in routine mental health agencies. Community Mental Health Journal, 2010;46:119–29.

[56] National Alliance on Mental Illness. Grading the States: a report on America's health care system for serious mental illness. Arlington: National Alliance on Mental Illness; 2006.

[57] Cunningham P, McKenzie K, Taylor E. The struggle to provide community-based care to low-income people with serious mental illness. Health Affairs 2006;25:694–705.

[58] Glied R, Frank R. Better but not best: recent trends in the well-being of the mentally ill. Health Affairs 2009;28:637–48.

[59] Goering P, Wasylenki D, Durbin J. Canada's mental health system. International Journal of Law and Psychiatry 2000;23:345–59.

[60] Rochefort D, Goering P. "More a link than division": how Canada has learned from US mental health policy. Health Affairs 1998;17:110–127.

[61] Jacobs P, Yim R, Ohinmaa A, Eng K, Dewa CS, Bland R, et al. Expenditures on mental health and addictions for Canadian provinces in 2003/04. The Canadian Journal of Psychiatry 2008;53:306–13.

[62] Standing Senate Committee on Social Affairs. Out of the shadows at last: transforming mental health, mental illness and addiction services in Canada. Ottawa: Government of Canada; 2006.

[63] Basauri VA. Cuba: Mental Health Care and Community Participation. In: Ameida JMC, Cohen A, editors. Innovative Mental Health Programs in Latin America and

the Caribbean. Washington: Pan American Health Organization (PAHO); 2008. pp. 67–79.

[64] Organizacion Panamericana de La Salud. Desarrollo de la Salud Mental en Panama. 1. Panama, Ministerio de Salud—Instituto Nacional de Salud Mental (INSEM). Serie de Salud Mental; 2007.

[65] World Health Organization. Integrating mental health into primary care: A global perspective. Geneva: WHO and World Organization of Family Doctors; 2008.

[66] World Health Organization. Ministry of Health of Costa Rica. Report of the Assessment of Mental Health Systems in Costa Rica using the WHO Assessment Instrument for Mental Health Systems (WHO-AIMS). Geneva: WHO; 2008.

[67] Collins PY. Argentina: Waving the mental health revolution banner—Psychiatric reform and community mental health in the province of Rio Negro. In: Ameida JMC, Cohen A, editors. Innovative Mental Health Programs in Latin America and the Caribbean. Washington: Pan American Health Organization (PAHO); 2008. pp. 1–32.

[68] Andreoli SB, Almeida-Filho N, Martin D, Mateus MD, Mari JJ. Is psychiatric reform a strategy for reducing the mental health budget? The case of Brazil. Revista Brasileira de Psiquiatria 2007;29:43–6.

[69] Mateus MD, Mari JJ, Delgado PG, Almeida-Filho N, Barrett T, Gerolin J, et al. The mental health system in Brazil: Policies and future challenges. International Journal of Mental Health Systems 2008;2:12.

[70] Henry C. Brazil: Two experiences with psychiatric deinstitutionalization, Campinas and Sobral. In: Ameida JMC, Cohen A, editors. Innovative Mental Health Programs in Latin America and the Caribbean. Washington: Pan American Health Organization (PAHO); 2008. pp. 33–43.

[71] Campos RT, Furtado JP, Passos E, Ferrer AL, Miranda L, Gama CA. Evaluation of the network of psychosocial care centers: between collective and mental health. Revista Panamericana de Salud Pública 2009;43:16–22.

[72] Figueiredo MD, Campos RO. [Mental health in the primary care system of Campinas, SP: network or spider's web?] Ciência & Saúde Coletiva 2009;14: 129–38.

[73] Araya R, Rojas G, Fritsch R, Gaete J, Rojas M, Simon G, et al. Treating depression in primary care in low-income women in Santiago, Chile: a randomised controlled trial. Lancet 2003;361:995–1000.

[74] Frammer CM. Chile: Reforms in National Mental Health Policy. In: Ameida JMC, Cohen A, editors. Innovative Mental Health Programs in Latin America and the Caribbean. Washington: Pan American Health Organization (PAHO); 2008. pp. 44–60.

[75] Bixby LR. [Assessing the impact of health sector reform in Costa Rica through a quasi-experimental study.] Revista Panamericana de Salud Pública 2004;15:94–103.

[76] Gallegos A, Montero F. Issues in Community-Based Rehabilitation for Persons with Mental Illness in Costa Rica. International Journal of Mental Health 1999;28:30–35.

[77] Arehart-Treichel J. Costa Rican psychiatrists proud of MH care system. Psychiatric News 2005;40:12.

[78] Aultman JM, Villegas EC. Ethical and social dilemmas surrounding community-based rehabilitation in Costa Rica. International Journal of Psychosocial Rehabilitation 2004;8. Epub. Available from: http://www.psychosocial.com/IJPR_8/Costa_Rica_Rehab.html.

[79] Hernandez BJ, Cabeza AA, Lopez F. La reorientación de la salud mental hacia la atención primaria en la provincia de Cienfuegos: Departamento de Salud Mental de la Provincia de Cienfuegos. In: Hernandez BJ, Cabeza AA, Lopez F, editors. Enfoques para um debate en salud mental. Havana: Ediciones Conexiones; 2002. pp. 109–37.

[80] Tablada HRC, Oliva RX. Demanda de atención institucional y psiquiatría comunitaria. Medisan 2002;6:11–17.

[81] Tablada HRC, Oliva RX. Estratégias de proyección comunitaria del hospital psiquiátrico su impacto en los indicadores hospitalarios. Revista del Hospital Psiquiátrico de la Habana 2006;3. Epub. Available from: http://www.revistahph .sld.cu/hph0106/hph01306.htm.

[82] McKenzie K. Jamaica: Community Mental Health Services. In: Ameida JMC, Cohen A, editors. Innovative Mental Health Programs in Latin America and the Caribbean. Washington: Pan American Health Organization (PAHO); 2008. pp. 79–92.

[83] Hickling FW. Community psychiatry and deinstitutionalization in Jamaica. Hospital & Community Psychiatry 1994;45:1122–6.

[84] Medina-Mora ME, Borges G, Muñoz CL, et al. Prevalencia de trastornos mentales y uso de servicios: Resultados de la encuesta nacional de epidemiologia psiquiátrica en México. Salud Mental 2003;26(4):1–16.

[85] Xavier M. Mexico: The Hidalgo experience: A new approach to mental health care. In: Ameida JMC, Cohen A, editors. Innovative Mental Health Programs in Latin America and the Caribbean. Washington: Pan American Health Organization (PAHO); 2008. pp. 97–111.

[86] Chandrasekhar CR. Development of community psychiatry. In: Bhugra D, Ranjith G, Patel V, editors. Handbook of Psychiatry: A South Asian Perspective. New Delhi: Byword Viva; 2005. pp. 422–33.

[87] Murthy SR. The national mental health programme: progress and problems. In: Agarwal SP, Goel DS, editors. Mental Health: An Indian Perspective 1946–2003. New Delhi: Directorate General of Health Services, Ministry of Health and Family Welfare; 2004. pp. 75–91.

[88] World Health Organization. The introduction of a mental health component into primary health care. Geneva: WHO; 1990.

[89] Patel V, Thara R. Meeting the mental health challenges: role of NGO initiatives. New Delhi: SAGE; 2003.

[90] Thara R, Islam A, Padmavati R. Beliefs about mental illness: a study of a rural South Indian community. International Journal of Mental Health 1998;27: 70–85.

[91] World Health Organization. WHO-AIMS report on mental health system in Bangladesh. Dhaka: WHO; 2007.

[92] Bangladeshi Mental Health Association Report; 2003.

[93] Dorji C. Achieving Gross National Happiness Through Community-Based Mental Health Services in Bhutan. Conf. Proc.; 2010.

[94] Chandrasekhar CR, Parthasarathy R. Community psychiatry. In: Vyas JN, Ahuja N, editors. Textbook of Post-Graduate Psychiatry, 2nd edition. New Delhi: Jaypee Brothers Medical Publishers; 1999. pp. 985–92.

[95] Padmavati R. Community mental health care in India. International Review of Psychiatry 2005;17:103–7.

[96] Patel V, Thara R. Meeting the Mental Health Needs of Developing Countries: NGO Innovations in India. London: Sage Publications; 2003.

[97] Chatterjee S, Chatterjee A, Jain S. Developing community based services for serious mental illness in a rural setting. In: Patel V, Thara R, editors. Meeting the Mental Health Needs of Developing Countries: NGO Innovations in India. New Delhi: Sage Publications; 2003. pp. 115–40.

[98] Nadkarni A. Outreach strategies in community mental health. In: Schizophrenia Research Foundation. Community Mental Health and Community Based Rehabilitation, Proceeding of SCARF-IDRC Seminar. Chennai, India; 1997.

[99] Thara R, Padmavati R. A community mental health program in rural Tamil Nadu. Asian Pacific Disability and Rehabilitation Journal 1999;10:34–5.

[100] Murthy RS. Rural psychiatry in developing countries. Psychiatric Services 1998;49:967–8.

[101] Regmi SK, Pokharel A, Ojha SP, Pradhan SN, Chapagain G. Nepal: Mental health country profile. International Review of Psychiatry 2004;16:142–9.

[102] Karim S, Saedd K, Rana MH. Pakistan: Mental health country profile. International Review of Psychiatry 2004;16:83–92.

[103] World Health Organization. WHO-AIMS Report on Mental Health System in Pakistan. Karachi: WHO; 2009.

[104] Wickramage K, Suveendran T, Mahoney J. Mental health in Sri Lanka: Evaluation of the impact of community support officers (CSO) in mental health service provision at district level. Colombo: WHO Country Office; 2009.

[105] Asia-Australia Mental Health (AAMH). Summary Report: Asia-Pacific Community Mental Health Development Project; 2008.

[106] Somasundaram DJ, van de Put WACM, Eisenbruch M, de Jong JTVM. Starting mental health services in Cambodia. Social Science & Medicine 1999;48:1029–46.

[107] Zwi AB, Silove D. Hearing the voices: mental health services in East-Timor. Lancet 2002;360:s45–6.

[108] Conde B. Philippines mental health country profile. International Review of Psychiatry 2004;16:159–66.

[109] Setiawan GP, Viora E. Disaster mental health preparedness plan in Indonesia. International Review of Psychiatry 2006;18:563–6.

[110] Htay H. Mental health and psychosocial aspects of disaster preparedness in Myanmar. International Review of Psychiatry 2006;18:579–85.

[111] Panyayong B, Pengjuntr W. Mental health and psychosocial aspects of disaster preparedness in Thailand. International Review of Psychiatry 2006;18:607–14.

[112] Prasetiyawan, Viora E, Maramis A, Keliat BA. Mental health model of care programmes after the tsunami in Aceh, Indonesia. International Review of Psychiatry 2006;18:559–62.

[113] Parameshvara DM. Malaysia mental health country profile. International Review of Psychiatry 2004;16:167–76.

[114] Ikebuchi E. Support of working life of persons with schizophrenia. Seishin Shinkeigaku Zasshi 2006;108:436–48.

[115] The National Addictions Management Service Homepage, http://www.nams.org.sg.

[116] Wei KC, Lee C, Wong KE. Community psychiatry in Singapore: An integration of community mental health services towards better patient care. The Hong Kong Journal of Psychiatry 2005;15:132–7.

[117] Pearson V. Community and culture: a Chinese model of community care for the mentally ill. International Journal of Social Psychiatry 1992;38:163–78.

[118] Phillips MR. Mental health services in China. Epidemiologia e Psichiatria Sociale 2000;9:84–8.

[119] Qiu F, Lu S. Guardianship networks for rural psychiatric patients: A non-professional support system in Jinshan County, Shanghai. British Journal of Psychiatry 1994;24:114–20.

[120] Phillips MR. The transformation of China's mental health services. China Journal 1998;39:1–36.

[121] Akiyama T, Chandra N, Chen CN, Ganesan M, Koyama A, Kua EE, et al. Asian models of excellence in psychiatric care and rehabilitation. International Review of Psychiatry 2008;20:445–51.

[122] Ito J, Oshima I, Nisho M, Kuno E. Initiative to build a community-based mental health system including assertive community treatment for people with sever mental illness in Japan. American Journal of Psychiatric Rehabilitation 2009;12:247–60.

[123] Yu J. Cost effectiveness of modified ACT program in Korea. World Association of Psychosocial Rehabilitation 10th Congress Bangalore, India; 2009.

[124] Yu J, Kim S, Ki S, Lee Y. Program for Assertive Community Treatment (PACT) in Korea: preliminary 7 months follow-up study. 161st American Psychiatric Association Annual Meeting Washington, DC; 2008.

[125] Fam J, Lee C, Lim BLLKK. Assertive community treatment (ACT) in Singapore: a 1-year follow-up study. Annals of the Academy of Medicine, Singapore 2007;36: 409–12.

[126] World Health Organization. WHO-AIMS Report on Mental Health System in the Republic of Azerbaijan. Baku, Azerbaijan: WHO and Ministry of Health; 2007.

[127] World Health Organization. European Health for All Database; 2009.

[128] Killion C, Cayetano C. Making mental health a priority in Belize. Archives of Psychiatric Nursing 2009;23:157–65.

[129] Furtado JP. [Needs evaluation of the sheltered homes in Brazilian public health system]. Ciência & Saúde Coletiva 2006;11:785–95.

[130] Oliveira GL, Caiaffa WT, Cherchiglia ML. [Mental health and continuity of care in healthcare centers in a city of Southeastern Brazil]. Revista Panamericana de Salud Pública 2008;42:707–16.

[131] Brasil Ministério da Saúde Coordenação Nacional de Saúde Mental. Saúde mental e atenção básica: o vínculo e o diálogo necessários, inclusão das ações de saúde mental na atenção básica. Brasília: Ministério da Saúde; 2005.

[132] Calipo PCB. Estudo descritivo do sistema de saúde mental do município de Santos no contexto da reforma da assistência psiquiátrica do sistema único de saúde do Brasil. Santos: Universidade Católica de Santos; 2008.

[133] Larrobla C, Botega NJ. [Psychiatric care policies and deinstitutionalization in South America]. Actas Españolas de Psiquiatría 2000;28:22–30.

[134] Araya R, Alvarado R, Minoletti A. Chile: An ongoing mental health revolution. Lancet 2009;374:597–8.

[135] Collins R, Green P. Community psychiatry and the Pan American Health Organization: The Jamaican experience. Bulletin of the Pan American Health Organization 1976;10:233–40.

[136] Jacob KS, Sharan P, Mirza I, Garrido-Cumbrera M, Seedat S, Mari JJ, et al. Mental health systems in countries: where are we now? Lancet 2007;370(9592):1061–77.

[137] World Health Organization. WHO-AIMS Report on Mental Health System in Republic of Korea. Gwacheon City, Republic of Korea: WHO and Ministry of Health and Welfare; 2007.

[138] Japan Ministry of Health Labour and Welfare. Patient Survey. Tokyo: Japan Ministry of Health, Labour and Welfare; 2005.

CHAPTER 5
Policies, plans, and programs

International and intercultural differences can play a significant role in shaping what mental health services are necessary and possible within local settings [1]. Nevertheless, in preparing this series of publications, we have been surprised to find that the most fundamentally important themes (in terms of both challenges and lessons learned) apply to many different countries and regions.

One challenge common to many countries worldwide is the difficulty of putting community mental health intentions into practice. We distinguish here between:

- National *policy* (or provincial or state policy in countries where health policy is set at that level): An overall statement of strategic intent (e.g. over a 5–10 year period) that gives direction to the whole system of mental health care. Such policies have been outlined for each region in Chapter 3.

- Implementation *plan*: An operational document setting out the specific steps needed to implement the national policy (e.g. what tasks are to be completed, by whom, by when, with which resources, and identifying the reporting lines and the incentives and sanctions if tasks are completed or not completed).

- Mental health *programs*: Specific plans either for a local area (e.g. a region or a district) or for a particular sector (e.g. primary care) that specify how one component of the overall care system should be developed.

According to the World Health Organization (WHO)'s Mental Health Atlas [2], 62.1% of countries worldwide had a mental health policy in place, and 70% had a mental health program in place, in 2005 (with 68 and 91% of the global population covered, respectively). Many of the countries without such policies were low- and middle-income countries (LAMICs). Even where comprehensive evidence-based mental health policies are in place, problems in implementing these policies are common [3, 4]. Consequently, the existence of mental health policies and legislation does not necessarily represent access to services in practice, and frequently access to mental health services is far more limited than is

Community Mental Health: putting policy into practice globally, First Edition. Graham Thornicroft, Maya Semrau, Atalay Alem, Robert E. Drake, Hiroto Ito, Jair Mari, Peter McGeorge, and R. Thara.
© 2011 John Wiley & Sons, Ltd. Published 2011 by John Wiley & Sons, Ltd.

prescribed by policies or legislation. Some of the reasons for this may include health staff not complying with policies due to difficulties in accepting and implementing changing roles [4], the lack of accessible evidence-based information or guidelines for health staff, insufficient funding mechanisms, inadequate training of health care personnel, the lack of mechanisms for training and coaching of health staff, poor supervision and support, and an overall lack of human resources [3].

South Asia is an example of a region where there have been great difficulties experienced in the implementation of mental health programs. Most countries in the region have few community mental health programs that stand the test of a critical appraisal, including a lack of adequate programs to train psychiatrists, psychiatric nurses, clinical psychologists, psychiatric social workers, and occupational therapists. Often these programs are sporadic, with no reenforcer sessions. Furthermore, many community mental health programs are put together in an ad hoc manner without much thought given to structure or function. Where projects are expected to last only a few years, this often does not seem to motivate professional management. Furthermore, there seems to be a lack of sensitivity to local social and cultural issues, and Western models are commonly thrust on an already unprepared and reluctant population.

Programs that do exist in the region are therefore often short-lived, with a few exceptions such as the National Mental Health Programme (NMHP) of India, which commenced in the 1980s, and has been heavily criticized. It was developed out of a concern for alternate care programs for the mentally ill and the initial experiences of organizing mental health care for the needy. Based on the principles of decentralization and destigmatization, the program aimed to integrate mental health care into primary care. Significant components of the program aimed to train health care personnel at all levels within primary health care centers, sensitizing policy planners to mental health issues, and promoting community participation in mental health service development.

Barriers to the implementation of the NMPH are outlined in Box 5.1. Critical factors identified as detriments to the NMHP's progress in India were a unidimensional, top-down program, poor funding, inadequate human resources, an uneven distribution of resources across states, and a lack of implementation of legal processes [5, 6]. Although the 11th five-year plan by the Government of India has more than doubled its funding for the NMHP, much of this remains unused. Partly this is due to the states not having had the personnel/trained manpower to fill all posts.

The absence of state-level plans has been another factor; only two or three states in India have their own plans for mental health. It was found that the entire program needed effective and efficient managers who could coordinate the program and work towards a beneficial outcome. Training

---

Box 5.1   Key barriers to the implementation of the National Mental Health Programme (NMHP) in India (according to Murthy 2004 [6]).

- Shortage of trained manpower in the field of mental health.
- Social stigma and lack of knowledge among psychiatric patients and their families.
- Negative attitudes of general practitioners, primary care physicians, and other specialists.
- NGO/voluntary organizations not finding this field attractive.
- Inadequate staff and infrastructure of mental hospitals and psychiatric wings in medical colleges.
- Uneven distribution of sparce resources, limiting the availability of mental health care to those living in urban areas.
- Inadequate funding for mental health, which remains a relatively low-priority area.

---

was erratic and inadequate, and the material for training was also un-satisfactory in some sites. Measures to monitor the program were not in place. Manpower constraints such as a lack of psychiatrists, psychologists, and other mental health staff compounded the problem further. There was also very little public–private partnership on the ground [7].

The Pacific Island Nations are another region where mental health programs have been scarce in the past. Although some Pacific Island Nations have mental health policies and/or plans in place (see Chapter 3), few have been resourced and governed in a way that is ensuring their implementation. A lack of training facilities and specialist staff has been one of the barriers to the implementation of mental health services.

This situation is changing however, with the inception of the Pacific Islands Mental Health Network (PIMHnet), which currently has 18 member countries (also see Chapter 4). PIMHnet's vision is "the people of Pacific Island countries enjoying the highest standards of mental health and well-being through access to effective, appropriate and quality mental health services and care". Its mission is "to facilitate and support cooperative and coordinated activities within and among member countries that contribute to sustainable national and sub-regional capacity in relation to mental health".

The overarching goals of the program are to build the capacity and capability of key people, and thereby their countries, and to support participants in planning for the development of mental health services in their countries. More specific objectives are:

- To identify and engage with individuals who have responsibilities towards the organization and development of mental health services.
- To work with participants to design country-based plans of action for developing an optimal mix of services.

- To design and implement projects which contribute to those plans, and which improve mental health service development, organization, and delivery.
- To provide coordinated and structured technical support to participants in terms of the development and implementation of action plans and associated projects.
- To create a network in the region, consisting of people who have responsibilities and/or expertise in relation to the organization and development of mental health services, and who may provide support for program participants.

Specific Pacific Island priorities include:

- Increasing the size and expertise of specialist workforces (almost universal).
- Improving training for the general health workforce (very common).
- Improving understanding and awareness of mental health in the community.
- Improving the organization and management of mental health services.
- Developing mental health policies and legislation.
- Developing/improving community-based care.

Considerable progress has been made by PIMHnet pilot member countries in identifying their mental health needs and resources, and in developing plans to address these needs. Twelve countries now have mental health human resource plans in place, designed to facilitate the development of human resources in ways that best meet the needs of individual countries.

In Latin American and Caribbean countries there has also been clear progress in the implementation of mental health programs. Table 5.1 summarizes the main findings of a literature search of studies on community mental health services in the region (see Table 1.1 in Chapter 1 for its methodology), many of which described or evaluated community mental health programs. For instance, specific programs to treat depression and to combat domestic violence were observed in Chile and Argentina. Furthermore, improvements in daily activities were observed for those patients transferred to sheltered homes in Mexico, and income-generating programs for patients discharged from psychiatric hospitals were carried out in Argentina and Brazil. In Argentina there were also successful experiences of integrating mental health with other sectors of society in small cities.

Moreover, the implementation of community mental health training had a positive impact in Argentina and Belize, increasing the number of mental health workers. Our literature search found that the hospitalization rate dropped between 5 and 50% in Argentina, Belize, Brazil, Cuba, and Jamaica. Moreover, the length of hospitalization was reduced, and the treatment coverage in community services increased for most countries.

Table 5.1 Summary of the main findings of mental health services research in Latin American and Caribbean countries.

	Main results
Argentina	• Integration between mental health and other non-health sectors: judges, police and mental health teams have created a network to combat domestic violence [8]. • Workshops on human rights and training in management of people in acute crisis on street [8]. • Creation of an income-generating program for people with mental disorders [8]. • Implementation of a residence program on community mental health, with an effect on decreasing the shortage of human resources in the regions of Rio Negro and Neuquén [8]. • After implementation of the Austral program in Neuquén, a reduction of hospitalization rate by 5%.
Belize	• Reduction in psychiatric hospital admissions. • Increase in the coverage and demand for treatment: outpatient services increased by 25% in 2002 [9].
Brazil	• Increase in the number of people receiving treatment for mental disorders in community mental health services in Santos [10], Campinas [11], and Sobral [9]. • Decrease in the number of psychiatric beds and in the rate of hospitalizations in Santos [12], Sobral [9], and Campinas [11]. • 20% of long-stay patients discharged from psychiatric hospitals transferred to sheltered homes. • Ministry of Health created the Return Home Programme, with financial benefits for patients discharged from psychiatric hospitals [10, 13]. • Patients involved in income-generating programs in Campinas [11] and Sobral.
Chile	• Increasing number of people receiving treatment in the public sector, from 40 000 attendances in 2003 to over 250 000 seen in 2008 [14]. • Increase in the number of people enrolled in a violence program: from 46 000 people in 1999 to 180 000 in 2003 [15]. • 29 000 subjects enrolled in a depression program in 2002 [16], and in 2004 the treatment coverage was 60% of the population [15]. • 6000 subjects treated with atypical antipsychotics in 2004 [15].
Cuba	• Reduction in the number of psychiatric beds in Havana [17]. • Between 1999 and 2004, a 25% reduction in hospitalization rates [17]. • Reduction in the number of long-stay patients in psychiatric hospitals, and a reduction in the length of hospitalizations [17].
Jamaica	• The number of patients hospitalized in Bellevue Hospital decreased by 58% (from 3094 patients in 1960 to 1296 in 1990). Admission rates decreased by 50% between 1971 and 1988 [18]. • 41 Mental Health Officers (MHOs) in the country, with an average caseload of 500 patients. Nearly 200 patients can be seen by an MHO monthly [19]. • 62% of 317 first-contact patients with schizophrenia treated at home [20].
Mexico	• The Ocaranza Asylum was closed and patients were transferred to 10 villas and 34 halfway houses. These patients had improved substantially in their daily activities when living in the community [21]. • Creation of a 30-bed acute psychiatric ward and a 24-hour emergency ward [21].

For example, more than 60% of first-contact patients with schizophrenia were treated at home in Jamaica.

In sum, there has been progress in the implementation of community mental health plans and programs in many countries worldwide, including in some areas where historically there has been a lack of such programs, as demonstrated by the example from the Pacific Nations. However, progress may often be slow or scarce in other areas, such as the South Asia region. Detailed and highly practical implementation plans (taking into account available resources) are therefore necessary across regions to enable effective community mental health care provision.

Key points in this chapter

- Many countries worldwide have experienced difficulties in putting community mental health intentions into practice, even in countries where dedicated national mental health policies are in place.
- Although well-planned mental health programs are still scarce in many countries worldwide, clear examples of these can be identified.
- Detailed and highly practical implementation plans and programs (in addition to mental health policies) are necessary across regions to enable effective community mental health care provision.
- Most countries appear to be better developed in terms of writing high-level strategic mental health policies than in terms of creating specific implementation plans that give details of who will be responsible for delivering which programs, with which resources, to which timescale, and with which lines of reporting and accountability.

References

[1] Saxena S, Thornicroft G, Knapp M, Whiteford H. Resources for mental health: scarcity, inequity, and inefficiency. Lancet 2007;370:878–89.
[2] World Health Organization. Mental Health Atlas, revised edition; 2005.
[3] Knapp M, McDaid D, Mossialos E, Thornicroft G. Mental Health Policy and Practice Across Europe: An Overview. In: Knapp M, McDaid D, Mossialos E, Thornicroft G, editors. Mental Health Policy and Practice Across Europe. Maidenhead: Open University Press; 2007. pp. 1–14.
[4] World Health Organization. Policies and Practices for Mental Health in Europe: Meeting the Challenges. WHO; 2008.
[5] Goel DS, Agarwal SP, Ichpujani RL, Shrivastava S. Mental Health 2003: The Indian Scene. In: Agarwal SP, Goel DS, editors. Mental Health: An Indian Perspective 1946–2003. New Delhi: Directorate General of Health Services, Ministry of Health and Family Welfare; 2004. pp. 3–24.
[6] Murthy SR. The national mental health programme: progress and problems. In: Agarwal SP, Goel DS, editors. Mental Health: An Indian Perspective 1946–2003.

New Delhi: Directorate General of Health Services, Ministry of Health and Family Welfare; 2004. pp. 75–91.

[7] Agarwal SP, Goel DS. Mental Health: An Indian Perspective 1946–2003. New Delhi: Directorate General of Health Services, Ministry of Health and Family Welfare; 2004.

[8] Collins PY. Argentina: Waving the mental health revolution banner—Psychiatric reform and community mental health in the province of Rio Negro. In: Ameida JMC, Cohen A, editors. Innovative Mental Health Programs in Latin America and the Caribbean. Washington: Pan American Health Organization (PAHO); 2008. pp. 1–32.

[9] World Health Organization and Wonca. Integrating mental health into primary care—A global perspective. Geneva: WHO and World Organization of Family Doctors; 2008.

[10] Calipo PCB. Estudo descritivo do sistema de saúde mental do município de Santos no contexto da reforma da assistência psiquiátrica do sistema único de saúde do Brasil. Santos: Universidade Católica de Santos; 2008.

[11] Henry C. Brazil: Two experiences with psychiatric deinstitutionalization, Campinas and Sobral. In: Ameida JMC, Cohen A, editors. Innovative Mental Health Programs in Latin America and the Caribbean. Washington: Pan American Health Organization (PAHO); 2008. pp. 33–43.

[12] Andreoli SB, Ronchetti Sde S, de Miranda AL, Bezerra CR, Magalhaes CC, Martin D, et al. [Utilization of community mental health services in the city of Santos, Sao Paulo, Brazil]. Cadernos de Saúde Pública 2004;20:836–44.

[13] Brasil Ministério da Saúde Secretaria de Atenção à Saúde CGdSM. Reforma psiquiátrica e política de saúde mental no Brasil. Conferência Regional de Reforma dos Serviços de Saúde Mental: 15 anos depois de Caracas. Brasília: Organización Panamericana de Salud; 2005.

[14] Araya R, Alvarado R, Minoletti A. Chile: An ongoing mental health revolution. Lancet 2009;374:597–8.

[15] Frammer CM. Chile: Reforms in National Mental Health Policy. In: Ameida JMC, Cohen A, editors. Innovative Mental Health Programs in Latin America and the Caribbean. Washington: Pan American Health Organization (PAHO); 2008. pp. 44–60.

[16] Larrobla C, Botega NJ. [Psychiatric care policies and deinstitutionalization in South America]. Actas Españolas de Psiquiatría 2000;28:22–30.

[17] Tablada HRC, Oliva RX. Estratégias de proyección comunitaria del hospital psiquiátrico su impacto en los indicadores hospitalarios. Revista del Hospital Psiquiátrico de la Habana 2006;3. Epub. Available from: http://www.revistahph .sld.cu/hph0106/hph01306.htm.

[18] McKenzie K. Jamaica: Community Mental Health Services. In: Ameida JMC, Cohen A, editors. Innovative Mental Health Programs in Latin America and the Caribbean. Washington: Pan American Health Organization (PAHO); 2008. pp. 79–92.

[19] Cunningham P, McKenzie K, Taylor E. The struggle to provide community-based care to low-income people with serious mental illness. Health Affairs 2006;25:694–705.

[20] Hickling FW, McCallum M, Nooks L, Rodgers-Johnson P. Outcome of first contact schizophrenia in Jamaica. The West Indian Medical Journal 2001;50:194–7.

[21] Xavier M. Mexico: The Hidalgo experience: A new approach to mental health care. In: Ameida JMC, Cohen A, editors. Innovative Mental Health Programs in Latin America and the Caribbean. Washington: Pan American Health Organization (PAHO); 2008. pp. 97–111.

CHAPTER 6
Scaling up services for whole populations

Treatment gap

A further challenge that needs to be addressed worldwide is the massive gap between population needs for mental health care (i.e. the true prevalence of mental illness) and what is actually provided in mental health care (i.e. treated prevalence) [1], highlighting the importance of scaling up services for whole populations.

Most people in the world who have mental illnesses receive no effective treatment [2–5]. For example, of all adults affected by mental illnesses, the proportion who are treated ranges from 30.5% in the USA [6], and 27% across Europe [7, 8], to less than 1% in Nigeria [3,9–12]. This "treatment gap" is increasingly appreciated worldwide [13–18].

It is notable that treatment rates differ substantially between physical and mental disorders worldwide. Table 6.1 shows that even in *high*-income countries treated prevalence rates for key mental disorders are much lower than those for physical disorders. Even more striking is that treatment rates for mental disorders in *high*-income countries are also substantially lower than treatment rates for physical disorders in *low*-income settings [10] (see Table 6.1).

Given this treatment gap, what service model for adults can help plan better care—and would be realistic—especially in relation to the vast differences in resources (largely in staff resources) available between high- and low-income settings, but also between high- and low-resource settings *within* countries [19, 20]?

The evidence concerning the substantial burden of mental disorders has not been translated into adequate investments in mental health care [16]. The treatment gap is particularly pronounced in low- and middle-income countries (LAMICs) (see Table 6.1), where commonly over 75% of people with mental disorders receive no treatment or care at all, and less than 2% of the health budget is spent on mental health [1]. Whilst the

Community Mental Health: putting policy into practice globally, First Edition. Graham Thornicroft, Maya Semrau, Atalay Alem, Robert E. Drake, Hiroto Ito, Jair Mari, Peter McGeorge, and R. Thara. © 2011 John Wiley & Sons, Ltd. Published 2011 by John Wiley & Sons, Ltd.

Table 6.1 Proportions of people with key physical and mental disorders who are treated, by high- versus low/middle-income country status (adapted from Ormel et al. 2008 [10]).

	High-income settings (% of cases which are treated)	Low- & middle-income settings (% of cases which are treated)
Physical disorders		
Diabetes	94%	77%
Heart disease	78%	51%
Asthma	65%	44%
Mental disorders		
Depression	29%	8%
Bipolar disorder	29%	13%
Panic disorder	33%	9%

high-income countries of the world have an average of 11 psychiatrists and 33 psychiatric nurses per 100 000 population (median figures), in low-income countries there are only 0.05 and 0.16, respectively [21] (also see Chapter 9). Furthermore, even within countries, the quality and level of services often vary greatly according to, for instance, patient group, location (with service provision usually being higher in urban areas), and socioeconomic factors [22].

For instance, only 57% of African countries report having community-based mental health care. Even though many policies support the decentralization of mental health services and the development of community-oriented services, actual implementation has been a great challenge across the African continent [23]. For most low-income African countries, achieving adequate population coverage with any kind of mental health care provision has been problematic, resulting in high treatment gaps for even the most severe mental disorders [15]. Similarly, in Latin American and Caribbean countries, the treatment gap for mental health is still a great challenge. The scarcity of mental health policies and care [24], combined with local factors such as the increasing rate of the aging population, as well as the effects of natural and human-made disasters, have contributed to the growing burden of mental disorders in the region, accounting for 18% of the total disease burden [25]. In the Australasia and South Pacific region, the major difficulties patients may have in accessing services have also been reported, as well as the disruptions experienced by them and their families in the continuity of care received. Similarly, up until recently most Pacific Island countries have not provided specialist training in mental health or addictions (the University of South Pacific being an exception), and there is considerable stigma towards mental illness [26]. As a result, access to contemporary psychiatric treatments such as medication has been extremely limited, as a result of both cost and limited laboratory facilities, as well as poor diagnoses and a lack of defined referral systems. As far as psychological treatments are concerned, these too have been extremely restricted. There is therefore a common theme across countries worldwide of a substantial number of patients not receiving the care they need.

Global mental health research

What is more, only 10% of global mental health research is directed to the health needs of the 90% of populations living in LAMICs, and only a fraction of this research activity is concerned with implementing and evaluating interventions and services [27]. For instance, a systematic review of published and grey literature in the Africa region of studies evaluating the implementation of community mental health care (the methodology is given in Box 1.1 in Chapter 1; a flow chart with details of the search results is shown in Figure 6.1) found that the vast majority of published mental

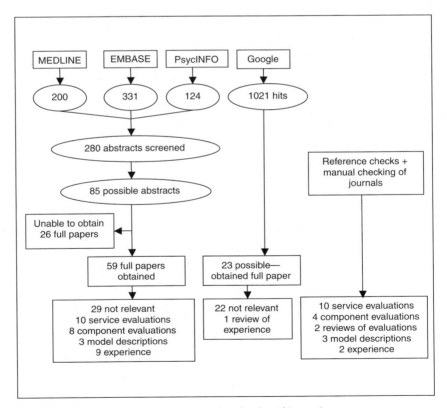

Figure 6.1 Search results of literature review for the Africa region.

Table 6.2 Locations of studies evaluating community mental health services in the Africa region.

	Number of publications	Number published since 2000
Botswana	3	0
Ghana	1	1
Guinea-Bissau	1	0
Lesotho	1	0
Nigeria	2	1
South Africa	17	8
Tanzania	2	1
Uganda	2	1
Zimbabwe	1	0
TOTAL	**29**	**12**

health service research in sub-Saharan Africa has been carried out in South Africa, an upper middle-income country. There was a conspicuous lack of published literature evaluating the implementation of community mental health care in low-income sub-Saharan African countries, particularly when considering more recent literature (since 2000) (see Table 6.2).

Evaluative studies of the implementation of community mental health services found during the literature search are summarized in Tables 6.3 and 6.4. Two reviews of evidence and experience arising from the implementation of community mental health care were also identified, both from South Africa [28, 29].

As illustrated in Table 6.5, only a minority of studies (n = 5) included a comparative element to their evaluation (either pre- compared to post-intervention, or compared to another service model), and only one randomized controlled trial (RCT) of an aspect of community mental health care was identified [30].

A previous critique of studies of mental health service development in South Africa highlighted similar gaps in the literature, and concluded that there was a particular need to develop, pilot, and formally evaluate (including cost-effectiveness) models of community mental health care rather than focus on descriptive studies of the challenges facing existing services [28]. Encouragingly, there are some evaluation studies of models for integration of mental health into primary health care now being conducted in several low-income African countries and due to report their findings in the near future, for example a cluster randomized trial to evaluate the effectiveness of training primary health care workers in mental health in Malawi [31] and an RCT in Kenya [32].

The identified studies in Africa have considered different models of community-based mental health care, looking at specialist assertive

Table 6.3 Studies evaluating multiple aspects of a community mental health care (CMHC) service in the Africa region.

Authors	CMHC evaluated	Model description	Study design	Main outcomes
South Africa				
Freed 1997 [39]	Community psychiatric clinic.	*Staff:* 2 psychiatric nurses, 1 social worker, weekly psychiatrist input. General nurses. TB outreach workers. *Target:* Community mental health care. *Activity:* Regular clinics, follow-up of discharged patients, home visits for defaulting patients.	Naturalistic follow-up over 6 months (random sample of n = 50 patients).	• 40% of patients (excluding mental retardation) able to resume work.
Lee et al. 1995 [43]	Community psychiatric clinic.	*Staff:* Community psychiatric nurse. *Target:* Psychiatric patients discharged from in-patient care. *Activity:* Monthly follow-up clinics held in primary health care (PHC) setting.	Retrospective review of clinical records (n = 488).	• Unnecessary polypharmacy in 9%. • Treatment inappropriate for diagnosis: 12–17%. • Rarely changed medication or discharged. Loss to follow-up over first year: 43–46%. • Patients with ≥3 relapses rarely referred.
Lee et al. 1999 [35]	Decentralized services to enable mental health care in PHC.	*Staff:* PHC nurses supported by monthly, 3-monthly, or 6-monthly visits from psychiatric nurses, psychologists, or psychiatrists. *Target:* Provide mental health (MH) care to community members with mental illness. *Activity:* Outpatient care for persons with mental illness. 16 general PHC clinics providing CMHC evaluated by study, chosen to reflect "good" (n = 7) and "indifferent" (n = 9) practice.	1) Quality of outpatient care. Review of random sample of n = 50 clinical records from each clinic.	• Good clinics diagnosed more conditions. • High levels of medication monotherapy. • Irregular attendance for 34–42% of patients. • Low defaulting rate: 15–18%. • Few patients discharged: 0–4%.

(Continued)

Table 6.3 Continued.

Authors	CMHC evaluated	Model description	Study design	Main outcomes
Lee et al. 1999 [63]			2) Impact of service change on PHC staff. Semistructured interviews (n = 29)	• 79% received training, 72% needed more. • 50% thought MH care added more stress. • 84% thought responsibility should be with MH workers. • Only 10% changed medication regimes.
Freeman et al. 1999 [40]			3) Social outcomes and patient perceptions. Semistructured interviews. Convenience sample. 114 attendees, 22 defaulters.	• 79% saw dispensing medication as main role. • Employment: 11% of black, 21% of white patients. • Impairment of social activities > personal care. • Majority (>90%) satisfied but >50% of black patients preferred long-stay hospital care. • Over 75% would like day services if available.
Freeman et al. 1999 [64]			4) Family burden. Convenience sample of family members: 63 attendees, 22 defaulters.	• 79–86% of patients lived with families. • Most happy to have patient staying at home. • Majority preferred long-stay hospital care. • High proportion wanted day care for patient.
Uys 2000 [36]	CMHC system in context of whole mental health service.	Different models of care in the different provinces. Evaluated any community-based mental health services, including hospital outpatient clinics and within PHC.	Comparison of public mental health services across three provinces: questionnaires for service providers and users; observation.	• Out of 13 quality standards, only one, with no information, was "community-based approach to care". • 40% of patients with enduring mental illness involved in rehabilitation. • In two provinces, psychosocial intervention documented in 10–22%.

Study	Topic	Description	Method	Findings
Petersen 2000 [37]	Mental health in PHC.	*Staff:* PHC nurses supported by monthly or bimonthly visits by specialist mental health team. *Target:* Mental health of community. *Activity:* Aiming to provide comprehensive mental health care integrated into PHC.	Ethnographic. In-depth interview of 6 PHC nurses, 9 patients with psychological disorder. Observation of clinical activities	• PHC nurses understand need for holistic care but provide largely biomedical care. • Factors from within the system and the macro-context militate against comprehensive mental health in PHC. • Need for paradigm shift.
Moosa & Jeenah 2008 [65]	Community mental health service.	*Staff:* Psychiatric nurses, psychiatrists. *Target:* Community mental health care. *Activity:* Weekly or monthly outpatient clinics conducted within PHC setting.	Retrospective audit of clinical records for year 2005.	• Narrow focus on medication. • Not comprehensive or accessible. • Short duration of appointments (8–10 minutes).
Botha et al. 2008 [66]	Assertive community team.	*Staff:* Medical officer, psychiatric nurse and senior social worker linked to hospital catchment area; 30–40 patients per key worker. *Target:* Revolving door patients. *Activity:* Monthly follow-up (including home visits) following inpatient admission.	Naturalistic follow-up (12 months) with mirror-image component.	• Reduction in duration of readmissions (100% of patients, n = 16).
Couper et al. 2006 [67]	Integrating MH into PHC.	PHC nurses providing bulk of mental health care in a "supermarket approach" (no specialist clinics), supported by specialist mental health services/mental health coordinator.	Quantitative study: Review of 142 clinical records and 584 clinic registers.	• No formal diagnosis in 44.4% of records. • Most patients on >1 medication (87.8%). • 36% of patients not seen within 6 months.

(Continued)

Table 6.3 Continued.

Authors	CMHC evaluated	Model description	Study design	Main outcomes
van Deventer 2008 [38]	Integrating MH into PHC.		Qualitative study. 5 focus group discussions with service users, 1 with mental health coordinators. 8 in-depth interviews with PHC workers.	• General satisfaction from patients and carers, but problems with communication, lack of continuity of care, long waiting times. • Mental health coordinators most negative. • PHC workers feel they do not have sufficient expertise, and problems individualizing treatment.
WHO & Wonca 2008 [33]	Ehlanzeni District integration of MH into PHC.	*Model 1:* Mental health nurse provides all MH care within PHC in separate weekly clinic. Other PHC workers trained to refer. *Model 2:* All PHC workers (medical officer and nurses) trained to manage MH problems.	Case study of best practice. Survey of staff and patients.	• Increased percentage of PHC clinics delivering mental health care (from 50 to 83%). • Amongst PHC workers, residual negative attitudes; 80% felt system could work, 62% thought number of health workers insufficient for successful integration. • Patients pleased with accessibility. In Model 1, more dissatisfaction about physical health care. • Model 2 less stigmatizing but with longer waits and concern about less continuity/quality of care.
	Moorreesburg District integration of MH into PHC.	*Model 3:* All PHC workers (medical officer and nurses) provide MH care in PHC. Monthly visit from MH nurse for supervision and training. Regional psychiatrist visits 3-monthly. Psychologist available.	Case study of best practice. Survey of staff.	• PHC workers generally satisfied with delivering MH care, appreciating specialist support. • Time and transport issues hinder outreach. • Social work services limited.

Petersen et al. 2009 [68]	Deinstitutionalization and integration of mental health in PHC.	Multicomponent community mental health system, focusing on district-level specialist mental health workers and integration of mental health service in PHC.	Quantitative questionnaire (WHO-AIMS) and qualitative study of key stakeholders: 34 in-depth interviews, 14 focus group discussions.	• Mental health coordinator and psychiatric nurses expanded to include non-mental health duties. • Minimal resources for prevention, promotion, training, and rehabilitation. • High turnover of PHC staff, loss of expertise in mental health care. • PHC workers do not feel competent to manage psychiatric problems. • Very low awareness of common mental disorders. • Psychosocial interventions limited to community health workers monitoring compliance.
Botswana Ben-Tovim 1983 [69], Ben-Tovim & Kundu 1982 [70]	Three rural regions implementing national program of integration of MH into PHC.	*Staff:* Psychiatric nurse or psychiatrist, PHC workers, family welfare educators (FWEs). *Target:* Mental health of community. *Activity:* Regular visits of specialist MH workers to PHC clinics to run joint clinics with PHC workers. Community mobilized by FWEs.	Descriptive cross-sectional evaluation.	• Community case-finding successful at increasing numbers treated in PHC. • Range of diagnoses as expected, expected relatively low identification of depressive psychosis. • About 25% lost to follow-up.

(Continued)

Table 6.3 Continued.

Authors	CMHC evaluated	Model description	Study design	Main outcomes
Guinea-Bissau				
de Jong 1996 [71]	National community mental health program.	*Staff:* PHC workers. *Target:* Mental health of community. *Activity:* 5 day training supported by supervision by specialist mental health workers (3-monthly in first year, annually thereafter).	Comparison of PHC worker MH skills pre- and post-intervention. Cost–benefit analysis.	• High turnover of PHC staff, so further training required. • Diagnostic sensitivity of PHC workers improved to 76% (specificity to 98%). • Supervision noted to be essential for success. • Patients/families reported improved symptoms. • Profitable cost–benefit ratio. • Sustainable from 1983 to 1994.
Nigeria				
Erinosho 1977 [72]	Aro community village program.	*Staff:* Next of kin stay with patient, village members live alongside, regular psychiatrist visits, collaboration with traditional healers. *Target:* Management of acutely unwell patients. *Activity:* Involvement in village activities, monitor medication. Psychotherapy/ECT as required.	Comparative, retrospective study. Aro mental hospital vs Aro community village program.	• No difference in readmission rates.

Tanzania Jablensky & Schulsinger 1991 [73], Bloch 1991 [74]	Integrating mental health into PHC.	*Staff:* PHC nurses trained for 1 month and supported by specialist mental health team at district and regional level, with district mental health coordinator. *Target:* Mental health at community level. *Activity:* Strengthened system at all levels. PHC workers to detect and treat priority conditions, and refer if necessary. Specialist mental health workers to provide longer-term care.	Attendance/referral patterns across mental health facilities in the pilot regions. Review of 694 clinical records.	• Program addresses an existing need, in line with that expected from epidemiological data. • Cost-effective when compared to hospital care. • Expected diagnostic spread of PHC workers. • Referral system operational. • Reportedly lowered inpatient admissions [83]. • Some inappropriate prescribing [84].
Uganda WHO & Wonca 2008 [33]	Integrating MH into PHC.	*Staff:* PHC workers, village health workers (volunteers), specialist MH workers, NGO. *Target:* Mental health of community. *Activity:* PHC workers identify and treat simple cases, manage emergencies and refer. Outreach and training from specialist MH workers.	Descriptive case study of effective implementation at pilot site.	• Marked increase in patients with mental health problems seen in PHC setting. • Increased referrals to regional rather than national psychiatric outpatient service. • Patients are satisfied with new service arrangement.
Multiple African centers BasicNeeds 2009 [75]	Community mental health program.	*Staff:* Community MH nurse/psychiatrist, PHC workers, community health workers (CHWs), traditional healers, religious leaders, service users. *Target:* Community mental health outreach. *Activity:* Regular clinics by psychiatric nurse/psychiatrist in outreach clinics, training of PHC nurses to deliver mental health care, community mobilization.	Case studies in Ghana, Kenya, Tanzania, Uganda. Focus groups, in-depth interviews, key informants, documentation analysis, and observation.	• Tanzania: Problem of fast turnover of PHC staff → mental health coordinator provided training. • Uganda: Service users taking on responsibility for case-finding help community outreach. • Problem of erratic supplies of medication. • Reliance on CHWs (volunteers) not sustainable. • Sustainability of outreach may be limited as parallel with PHC system in some centers.

Table 6.4 Studies evaluating a component of community mental health care (CMHC) in the Africa region.

Authors	Aspect of CMHC evaluated	Model description	Study design	Main outcomes
South Africa				
Gillis et al. 1989 [30]	Post-discharge medication adherence.	*Staff:* Psychiatric nurses. *Target:* Admitted patients. *Activity:* Compared four groups: (i) ward staff giving medication information; (ii) as (i) but reinforced by pharmacist; (iii) as (i) but also discussion with psychiatric nurse; (iv) as (i) but also home visit from psychiatric nurse in first week.	Randomized controlled trial (n = 50 in each arm).	• Home visit markedly more effective at improving adherence compared to all other intervention arms (64% vs 37% or less).
Gillis et al. 1990 [76]	Post-discharge home-visiting program.	*Staff:* Psychiatric nurses. *Target:* Readmitted patients. *Activity:* Pre-discharge meeting with patient, then home visits as indicated.	Mirror image design with 12-month follow-up. n = 50.	• Decreased days in hospital (total of 3714 vs 1850). • 31.5% reduction in readmissions. • 39.0% improvement in clinic attendance.
Koch & Gillis 1991 [77]	Post-discharge mental health clinic.	*Staff:* Specialist mental health (MH) workers. *Target:* Recently admitted patients. *Activity:* Outpatient care in community setting, with no home visits/outreach service.	Naturalistic follow-up (12 months) of 136 patients.	• Practical difficulties contributing to nonattendance. • Nonattendance associated with increased risk of readmission: 67.5% vs 20% of regular attendees.
Petersen & Pillay 1997 [41]	Referral system to primary health care (PHC)	*Staff:* Community health workers (CHWs) (volunteers). *Target:* Patients in the community needing referral for mental health assessment/treatment. *Activity:* Completion of referral form and information sent back from PHC to referrer.	File audit of referrals (n = 72) over a 5-month period.	Effectiveness of referral system reduced by: • Lack of cooperation from PHC workers. • Ambiguity of CHW role, leading to poor motivation. • Traditional healer the CHW with most referrals and back-referrals. • Referrals made directly to specialist mental health services often inappropriate.

Sokhela & Uys 1998 [45]	Rehabilitation in PHC.	*Staff:* PHC nurses. *Target:* Patients with severe and enduring mental illness. *Activity:* PHC nurses given 10 days of training in provision of rehabilitation.	Naturalistic, follow-up (12 and 18 months) of PHC nurse case documentation post-training in 6 clinics.	• >65% documented target symptom, developed plan for patient and family, set rehabilitation goals and steps to achieve goals, increasing after refresher training.
Sokhela 1999 [78]	Effectiveness of PHC worker training.	*Staff:* Selected PHC nurses (2 per clinic). *Target:* Enable to diagnose, treat, and appropriately refer selected psychiatric conditions. *Activity:* Training for 63.5 hours, largely practical.	Patient records completed by 26 nurses (6 clinics) after completing training; reviewed by psychiatrists. Cross-sectional. n = 211.	• Improved patient vocational rehabilitation. • Complete psychiatric histories in 89%. • Diagnosis correct in 63%. • Appropriate prescription: 92% for emergency medication, 60% for long-term medication.
Richards et al. 2007 [79]	Maintaining patients in follow-up.	*Staff:* Community-based workers (volunteers). *Target:* Patients defaulting on appointments. *Activity:* Tracing defaulting patients.		• 57% of defaulting patients returned to clinic.
Zimbabwe Buchan & Hudson 1975 [80]	Post-discharge follow-up.	*Staff:* Psychiatric nurse attending PHC every other month to support medical officer, medical assistant, and health assistant. *Target:* Post-discharge patients. *Activity:* Regular clinic review and outreach.	Evaluating impact of new follow-up clinics (n = 25) compared to district with no follow-up service. 1-year follow-up. n = 406.	• No effect on readmission rate compared to other district. • Never attended: 64% rural, 46% urban. • Still in follow-up after 1 year: 26% vs 38%. • Attending all appointments: 5% vs 16%.

(Continued)

Table 6.4 Continued.

Authors	Aspect of CMHC evaluated	Model description	Study design	Main outcomes
Lesotho				
Meursing & Wankiiri 1988 [42]	PHC nurse adherence to clinical flow charts.	*Staff:* PHC nurses. *Target:* Appropriate management plan. *Activity:* 13 hours of training in use of clinical flow charts.	Evaluation of PHC nurse management plans for 105 patients, compared to MH specialists.	• 74% of patients identified and treated correctly. • Errors in flow charts accounted for almost half of mistakes.
Botswana				
Kgosidintsi 1996 [81]	Community mental health nurse role in PHC.	*Staff:* Community mental health nurse in PHC. *Target:* Mental health in community and PHC patients. *Activity:* Responsible for prevention and promotion activities, supervising general PHC workers, and coordinating delivery of MH care in PHC.	Mixed qualitative–quantitative study. Semistructured interviews with 9 nurses and 25 carers, observation, and documentary analysis.	• Role of community MH nurse largely technical, limited to monitoring mental states, prescribing and administering depot medication. Mostly clinic-based. • Carers articulated need for greater support in order to be able to maintain patients in their homes, e.g. periodic respite care.
Nigeria				
Eaton & Agomoh 2008 [82]	Community-based awareness program.	*Staff:* Village-based health workers (volunteers). *Target:* Community mental health. *Activities:* 1-week training to increase awareness, reduce stigma, promote rights.	Naturalistic, prospective study.	• Significant increase in new patient attendances at PHC clinics. • Increase waned with time, but remained higher than baseline.

Table 6.5 Types of studies evaluating community mental health care
in the Africa region.

	Number
Randomized controlled trial	1
Pre–post evaluation	3
Non-randomized comparative	1
Descriptive quantitative	16
Multimethod descriptive case study	3
Qualitative study	3
TOTAL	**27**

outreach teams, the benefits of home visits by mental health nurses in improving treatment adherence and reducing readmissions, and variations on the integration of mental health into primary health care. For example: joint clinics between primary health workers and mental health nurses, mental health nurses working in a primary health care setting, and primary health workers providing the bulk of mental health care, with varying degrees of specialist mental health support. Little is known about the relative merits of these different approaches, as few studies have directly compared their effectiveness, with the exception of the WHO South Africa case studies [33].

Much of the focus of studies in the Africa region has been on the quality of mental health care provided within primary health care, as well as on the skills, knowledge, and attitudes of primary health care workers in relation to the diagnosis and management of mental disorders. Previously, studies of the effectiveness of training primary health care workers to deliver mental health care have been criticized for relying on self-reports from primary health care workers (subject to social desirability bias) and failing to look at the sustainability of the effect of training [34]. By examining case records kept by primary health care workers (e.g. [35]), some of the subjectivity of assessment can be overcome, although documented practice may not fully accord with actual clinical practice.

Some studies incorporating observational methods have yielded important insights [36, 37], for example revealing that the emotional work required for dealing with patients with mental disorders may contribute to primary health care workers preferring to operate in a task-orientated biomedical model of care rather than the more holistic model envisaged by the primary health care model [37]. Although several studies have included evaluations of the levels of satisfaction with services expressed by patients and their families [38], and two studies have considered patients' social outcomes [39, 40], no study was identified that evaluated patients' clinical outcomes using standardized diagnostic or symptom scales, and no study looked at patient experience of side-effects of medication or physical health parameters. This is much in keeping with the findings from Cohen's review, published ten years ago [34].

Aside from evaluations of the effectiveness of training primary health care workers, only a handful of studies in the Africa region have attempted to evaluate the individual service processes necessary for the successful implementation of community mental health care, for example by considering the effectiveness of referral networks [41] and clinical protocols [42]. No studies were identified examining the quality and quantity of supervision required to enable adequate delivery of mental health care by primary health care workers, despite the recognized importance of supervision for the success of integration of mental health into primary health care [34]. The finding that even mental health nurses seem reluctant to revise diagnoses, change medication protocols, and proactively discharge patients from follow-up [43] underlines the importance of evaluating supervision arrangements.

There is also an absence of studies in the Africa region evaluating the effectiveness of psychosocial interventions delivered within the constraints of the primary health care setting. Group interpersonal therapy has been shown to be effective for persons with depressive disorder in a rural Ugandan setting [44], but the intervention was delivered by an NGO in parallel with the health system. One exception is a study evaluating the incorporation of psychosocial rehabilitation for those with severe mental illness into the role of primary health care nurses [45]. Understanding whether similar brief interventions are feasible or effective in primary health care settings, or whether primary health care workers can collaborate with NGOs and community-based organizations to provide such interventions, is an important topic for future research in the Africa region [46–48].

The picture is similar in the East and South-East Asia region, where there have been very few research studies published on regional community mental health services (at least ones published in English). When conducting a MEDLINE search for the region using the term "community mental health" (limited to English publications), of the 383 studies originally retrieved from this search, 125 were identified as relevant. Of these, 16% dealt with schizophrenia. Nearly half of the literature (46%) had been written before 2000. Only seven (6%) were RCT trials, four (3%) were non-randomized trials, 29 (23%) were service evaluations, 22 (18%) were surveys including epidemiological studies, and more than half (50%) were descriptive reports and "non-research" papers. Two-thirds of the studies were generated in China and Japan. About half of the studies from China were from Hong Kong.

Estimating needs and priority-setting

Methods to estimate resource needs are also necessary in scaling up services. A systematic methodology for setting priorities in child health research has been developed, taking into consideration that interventions should be effective, sustainable, and affordable in order to reduce the burden of disease [49]. A similar methodology was applied by the *Lancet* Global Mental Health Group, which focused on four groups of disorders whilst setting priorities for global mental health research: depressive, anxiety, and other common mental disorders; alcohol- and other substance-abuse disorders; child and adolescent mental disorders; and schizophrenia and other psychotic disorders [51]. It was recommended that interventions should be delivered by non-mental health professionals within existing routine care settings, and specialists should play a role in capacity-building and supervision [52].

A comprehensive review of packages of care for six leading neuropsychiatric disorders—attention deficit hyperactivity disorder (ADHD), alcohol abuse, dementia, depression, epilepsy, and schizophrenia—has also recently been proposed as a means to extend treatment in LAMICs [53–57]. A survey of the availability and feasibility of various treatments for the most prevalent mental disorders in the various age groups has recently been carried out by the World Psychiatric Association (WPA) among its member societies [58].

An extensive set of treatment guidelines, also suitable for LAMICs, was published by the World Health Organization (WHO) in 2010 as a part of its Mental Health Global Action Programme (mhGAP). The Department of Mental Health and Substance Abuse at the WHO recognized the importance of this challenge by launching the mhGAP in 2008 [59]. The first major product of this program was the mhGAP Implementation Guide (MIG) [59–61]. The MIG contains case finding and treatment guidelines for nine important categories of mental and neurological disorders that are common in low-income settings and which have a major public health impact: depression, psychoses, epilepsy/seizures, developmental disorders, behavior disorders, dementia, alcohol-use disorders, drug-use disorders, and self-harm/suicide. The MIG is based upon 93 thorough literature reviews using the Grading of Recommendations Assessment, Development and Evaluation (GRADE) methodology [58, 59, 62], and is available from http://www.who.int/mental_health/evidence/mhGAP_intervention_guide/en/index.html.

Key points in this chapter

- There is a vast gap between population needs for mental health care and what is actually provided in mental health care.
- Although this is a recurrent theme across countries, the mental health treatment gap is particularly pronounced in LAMICs.
- Research concerned with the implementation and evaluation of community mental health services is scarce, especially in LAMICs. More research is needed across regions to enable the implementation of evidence-based interventions and programs that are accessible to whole populations.
- There have been various documents published recently outlining comprehensive interventions/packages of care, including publications by the *Lancet* Global Mental Health Group, PLOS Medicine Series, and the WHO's mhGAP.

References

[1] World Health Organization. Mental Health Gap Action Programme—Scaling Up Care for Mental, Neurological, and Substance Use Disorders. 2008.

[2] Thornicroft G. Most people with mental illness are not treated. Lancet 2007;370(9590):807–8.

[3] Wang PS, Aguilar-Gaxiola S, Alonso J, Angermeyer MC, Borges G, Bromet EJ, et al. Use of mental health services for anxiety, mood, and substance disorders in 17 countries in the WHO world mental health surveys. Lancet 2007;370(9590):841–50.

[4] Kessler RC, Guilar-Gaxiola S, Alonso J, Chatterji S, Lee S, Ormel J, et al. The global burden of mental disorders: an update from the WHO World Mental Health (WMH) surveys. Epidemiol Psichiatr Soc 2009;18(1):23–33.

[5] Patel V, Maj M, Flisher AJ, DE Silva MJ, Koschorke M, Prince M. Reducing the treatment gap for mental disorders: a WPA survey. World Psychiatry 2010;9(3):169–76.

[6] Kessler RC, Demler O, Frank RG, Olfson M, Pincus HA, Walters EE, et al. Prevalence and treatment of mental disorders, 1990 to 2003. N Engl J Med 2005;352(24):2515–23.

[7] Wittchen HU, Jacobi F. Size and burden of mental disorders in Europe—a critical review and appraisal of 27 studies. Eur Neuropsychopharmacol 2005;15(4):357–76.

[8] Alonso J, Codony M, Kovess V, Angermeyer MC, Katz SJ, Haro JM, et al. Population level of unmet need for mental healthcare in Europe. Br J Psychiatry 2007;190:299–306.

[9] Kohn R, Saxena S, Levav I, Saraceno B. Treatment gap in mental health care. Bull World Health Organ 2004;82:858–66.

[10] Ormel J, Petukhova M, Chatterji S, guilar-Gaxiola S, Alonso J, Angermeyer MC, et al. Disability and treatment of specific mental and physical disorders across the world. Br J Psychiatry 2008;192:368–75.

[11] Demyttenaere K, Bruffaerts R, Posada-Villa J, Gasquet I, Kovess V, Lepine JP, et al. Prevalence, severity, and unmet need for treatment of mental disorders in the World Health Organization World Mental Health Surveys. JAMA 2004;291(21):2581–90.

[12] Wang P, Kessler R, et al. Treated and untreated prevalence of mental disorder. In: Thornicroft G, Szmukler G, Mueser K, Drake RE, editors. Oxford Textbook of Community Mental Health. Oxford: Oxford University Press; 2011.

[13] Prince M, Patel V, Saxena S, Maj M, Maselko J, Phillips MR, et al. No health without mental health. Lancet 2007;370(9590):859–77.

[14] Patel V, Araya R, Chatterjee S, Chisholm D, Cohen A, De SM, et al. Treatment and prevention of mental disorders in low-income and middle-income countries. Lancet 2007;370(9591):991–1005.

[15] Saxena S, Thornicroft G, Knapp M, Whiteford H. Resources for mental health: scarcity, inequity, and inefficiency. Lancet 2007;370(9590):878–89.

[16] Jacob KS, Sharan P, Mirza I, Garrido-Cumbrera M, Seedat S, Mari JJ, et al. Mental health systems in countries: where are we now? Lancet 2007;370(9592): 1061–77.

[17] Saraceno B, van Ommeren M, Batniji R, Cohen A, Gureje O, Mahoney J, et al. Barriers to improvement of mental health services in low-income and middle-income countries. Lancet 2007;370(9593):1164–74.

[18] Chisholm D, Flisher AJ, Lund C, Patel V, Saxena S, Thornicroft G, et al. Scale up services for mental disorders: a call for action. Lancet 2007;370(9594):1241–52.

[19] Thornicroft G, Tansella M. Better Mental Health Care. Cambridge: Cambridge University Press; 2009.

[20] Thornicroft G, Tansella M. What are the arguments for community-based mental health care? Copenhagen: WHO Regional Office for Europe; 2003.

[21] World Health Organization. Mental Health Atlas, revised edition. 2005.

[22] World Health Organization. The World Health Report 2001—Mental Health: New Understanding, New Hope. 2001.

[23] Kigozi F. Integrating mental health into primary health care: Uganda's experience. South African Psychiatry Review 2007;10(1):17–19.

[24] Kohn R, Levav I, de Almeida JM, Vicente B, Andrade L, Caraveo-Anduaga JJ, et al. Mental disorders in Latin America and the Caribbean: a public health priority. Revista Panamericana de Salud Pública. 2005;18:229–240.

[25] Hyman S, Chisholm D, Kessler R, Patel V, Whiteford H. Mental Disorders. In: Jamison DT, Breman JG, Measham AR, Alleyne G, Claeson M, Evans DB, et al., editors. Disease Control Priorities in Developing Countries. Geneva: The World Bank and WHO; 2006. pp. 605–25.

[26] Hughes F, Finlayson M, Firkin MP, Funk M, Drew N, Barrett T, et al. Situational Analysis of Mental Health Needs and Resources in Pacific Island Countries. Centre for Mental Health Research PaSD, Geneva: WHO; 2005.

[27] Saxena S, Paraje G, Sharan P, Karam G, Sadana R. The 10/90 divide in mental health research: trends over a 10-year period. British Journal of Psychiatry 2006;188:81–2.

[28] Thom R. Mental health services research review final report (Grant 256/00). South Africa: Health Systems Trust; 2003.

[29] Mkhize N, Kometsi M. Community access to mental health services: lessons and recommendations. 2008. Report No.: Chapter 7.

[30] Gillis LS, Koch A, Joyl M. Improving compliance in Xhosa psychiatric patients. South African Medical Journal 1989;76(5):205–8.

[31] Kauye F. Primary health workers' training in mental health and its impact on service delivery in the Southern region of Malawi. World Psychiatric Association Regional Meeting: Scaling up and reaching down—addressing unmet need for services. Abuja, Nigeria: African Association of Psychiatrists and Allied Professions Conference; 2009.

[32] Jenkins R, Kiima D, Njenga F, Okonji M. Increasing access to mental health services in Kenya a national primary care training programme. Abuja, Nigeria: African Association of Psychiatrists and Allied Professions; 2009.

[33] WHO and Wonca. Integrating mental health into primary care: a global perspective. Geneva: WHO and World Organization of Family Doctors; 2008.

[34] Cohen A. The effectiveness of mental health services in primary care: the view from the developing world. Geneva: WHO; 2001.

[35] Lee T, Freeman M, Vivian W. Evaluation of mental health services in the free state. Part I. Quality of outpatient care. South African Medical Journal 1999;89(Spec. Issue 1 March).

[36] Uys LR. The evaluation of public psychiatric services in three provinces of South Africa. South African Medical Journal 2000;90(6):626–30.

[37] Petersen I. Comprehensive integrated primary mental health care for South Africa. Pipedream or possibility? Social Science & Medicine 2000;51(3):321–34.

[38] van Deventer C, Couper I, Wright A, Tumbo J, Kyeyune C. Evaluation of primary mental health care in North West province: a qualitative view. South African Journal of Psychiatry 2008;14(4):136–40.

[39] Freed ED. A community psychiatric programme for Soweto: report on a pilot study. South African Medical Journal 1979;55(17):679–82.

[40] Freeman M, Lee T, Vivian W. Evaluation of mental health services in the free state. Part III. Social outcome and patient perceptions. South African Medical Journal 1999;89(Spec. Issue 1 March).

[41] Petersen I, Pillay YG. Facilitating community mental health care in South Africa: the role of community health workers in the referral system. South African Medical Journal 1997;87(11):1621–6.

[42] Meursing K, Wankiiri V. Use of flow-charts by nurses dealing with mental patients: an evaluation in Lesotho. Bulletin of the World Health Organization 1988; 66(4):507–14.

[43] Lee T, Prince M, Allwood CW. The outpatient care of psychiatric patients in a rural area: Mhala district, Northern Transvaal. South African Medical Journal 1995;85(6):571–7.

[44] Bolton P, Bass J, Neugebauer R, Verdeli H, Clougherty KF, Wickramaratne P, et al. Group interpersonal psychotherapy for depression in rural Uganda. JAMA 2003;289(23):3117–24.

[45] Sokhela NE, Uys LR. The integration of the rehabilitation of psychiatric patients into the primary health care system. Curationis 1998;21(4):8–13.

[46] Flisher AJ, Lund C, Funk M, Banda M, Bhana A, Doku V, et al. Mental health policy development and implementation in four African countries. J Health Psychol 2007 May;12(3):505–16.

[47] Petersen I, Bhana A, Campbell-Hall V, Mjadu S, Lund C, Kleintjies S, et al. Planning for district mental health services in South Africa: a situational analysis of a rural district site. Health Policy Plan 2009 Mar;24(2):140–50.

[48] Campbell-Hall V, Petersen I, Bhana A, Mjadu S, Hosegood V, Flisher AJ. Collaboration between traditional practitioners and primary health care staff in South

Africa: developing a workable partnership for community mental health services. Transcult Psychiatry 2010 Sep;47(4):610–28.

[49] Rudan I, Chopra M, Kapiriri L, Gibson J, Ann Lansang M, Carneiro I, et al. Setting priorities in global child health research investments: universal challenges and conceptual framework. Croation Medical Journal 2008;49(3):307–17.

[50] Patel V, Araya R, Chowdhary N, King M, Kirkwood B, Nayak S, et al. Detecting common mental disorders in primary care in India: a comparison of five screening questionnaires. Psychol Med 2008 Feb;38(2):221–8.

[51] Lancet Global Mental Health Group. Global Mental Health 6. Scale up services for mental disorders: a call for action. Lancet 2007;370(9594):1241–52.

[52] Patel V. The future of psychiatry in low- and middle-income countries. Psychological Medicine 2009;39:1759–62.

[53] Patel V, Thornicroft G. Packages of care for mental, neurological, and substance use disorders in low- and middle-income countries: PLoS Medicine Series. PLoS Med 2009 Oct;6(10):e1000160.

[54] Patel V, Simon G, Chowdary N, Kaaya S, Araya R. Packages of care for depression in low- and middle-income countries. PLoS Medicine 2009;6(10):e1000159.

[55] Mbuba CK, Newton CR. Packages of care for epilepsy in low- and middle-income countries. PLoS Medicine 2009;6(10):e1000162.

[56] Benegal V, Chand PK, Obot IS. Packages of care for alcohol use disorders in low- and middle-income countries. PLoS Medicine 2009;6(10):e1000170.

[57] de Jesus MJ, Razzouk D, Thara R, Eaton J, Thornicroft G. Packages of care for schizophrenia in low- and middle-income countries. PLoS Med 2009 Oct;6(10):e1000165.

[58] Patel V, Maj M, Flisher AJ, de Silva MJ, Koschorke M, Prince M, et al. Reducing the treatment gap for mental disorders: A WPA survey. World Psychiatry 2010; 9(3):169–76.

[59] World Health Organization. mhGAP Intervention Guide. Geneva: WHO; 2010.

[60] Hill S, Pang T. Leading by example: a culture change at WHO. Lancet 2007; 369(9576):1842–4.

[61] World Health Organization. WHO Handbook for guideline development. 2009. Available from http://www.searo.who.int/LinkFiles/RPC_Handbook_Guideline _Development.pdf.

[62] World Health Organization. mhGAP: Mental Health Gap Action Programme: scaling up care for mental, neurological and substance use disorders. Geneva: WHO; 2008.

[63] Lee T, Freeman M, Vivian W. Evaluation of mental health services in the free state. Part II. Training, attitudes and practices of generalist and psychiatric nurses. South African Medical Journal 1999;89(Spec. Issue 1 March).

[64] Freeman M, Lee T, Vivian W. Evaluation of mental health services in the free state. Part IV. Family burden and perspectives. South African Medical Journal 1999;89(Spec. Issue 1 March).

[65] Moosa MYH, Jeenah FY. Community psychiatry: An audit of the services in southern Gauteng. South African Journal of Psychiatry 2008;14(2):36–43.

[66] Botha U, Koen L, Oosthuizen P, Hering L. Assertive community treatment in the South African context. African Journal of Psychiatry 2008;11(4):272–5.

[67] Couper I, Wright A, van Deventer C, Kyeyune C, Tumbo J, Musonda J, et al. Evaluation of primary mental health care in north west province: final report. Johannesburg: University of Witwatersrand; 2006.

[68] Petersen I, Bhana A, Campbell-Hall V, Mjadu S, Lund C, Kleintjies S, et al. Planning for district mental health services in South Africa: a situational analysis of a rural district site. Health, Policy and Planning 2009;24(2):140–50.

[69] Ben-Tovim DI. A psychiatric service to the remote areas of Botswana. British Journal of Psychiatry 1983;142:199–203.

[70] Ben-Tovim DI, Kundu P. Botswana: Integration of psychiatric care with primary health care. Lancet 1982;320(8301):757–8.

[71] de Jong TVM. A comprehensive public mental health programme in Guinea-Bissau: a useful model for African, Asian and Latin-American countries. Psychological Medicine 1996;26:97–108.

[72] Erinosho OA. Mental health delivery-systems and post-treatment performance in Nigeria. Acta Psychiatrica Scandinavica 1977;55(1):1–9.

[73] Jablensky A, Schulsinger F. The national mental health programme in the United Republic of Tanzania: A report from WHO and DANIDA. Acta Psychiatrica Scandinavica 1991;83(S364):1–132.

[74] Bloch M. Treatment of psychiatric patients in Tanzania. Chapter 10. Acta Psychiatrica Scandinavica Supplementum 1991;83(S364):122–9.

[75] BasicNeeds. Community mental health practice: seven essential features for scaling up in low- and middle-income countries. Bangalore; 2009.

[76] Gillis LS, Koch A, Joyi M. The value and cost-effectiveness of a home-visiting programme for psychiatric patients. South African Medical Journal 1990;77(6): 309–10.

[77] Koch A, Gillis LS. Non-attendance of psychiatric outpatients. South African Medical Journal 1991;80(6):289–91.

[78] Sokhela NE. The integration of comprehensive psychiatric/mental health care into the primary health system: diagnosis and treatment. Journal of Advanced Nursing 1999;30(1):229–37.

[79] Richards DA, Bradshaw TJ, Mairs H, Ricks E, Strumpher J, Williams N, et al. Can community volunteers work to trace patients defaulting from scheduled psychiatric clinic appointments? South African Medical Journal 2007;97(10):946–7.

[80] Buchan T, Hudson G. Psychiatric follow-up services in Matabeleland. South African Medical Journal 1975;49(1):21–6.

[81] Kgosidintsi A. The role of the community mental health nurse in Botswana: the needs and problems of carers of schizophrenic clients in the community. Curationis 1996;19(2):38-42.

[82] Eaton J, Agomoh AO. Developing mental health services in Nigeria: the impact of a community-based mental health awareness programme. Social Psychiatry and Psychiatric Epidemiology 2008;43(7):552–8.

[83] Kilonzo GP, Simmons N. Development of mental health services in Tanzania: a reappraisal for the future. Social Science & Medicine 1998; 47(4):419–28.

[84] Kempinski R. Mental health and primary health care in Tanzania. Acta Psychiatrica Scandinavica 1991; 83(S364):112–21.

CHAPTER 7

Stigma, discrimination, and community awareness about mental illnesses

Introduction

The effects of stigmatization upon people with mental illness are common and profoundly socially excluding, and so constitute unethical global barriers to full social participation.

Understanding stigma and discrimination

"Stigma" (plural stigmata) has been used to refer to an indelible dot left on the skin after stinging with a sharp instrument, sometimes to identify vagabonds or slaves [1, 2]. Recently stigma has come to mean "any attribute, trait or disorder that marks an individual as being unacceptably different from the 'normal' people with whom he or she routinely interacts, and that elicits some form of community sanction" [3–5].

A sizeable literature now refers to stigma [3, 6–17]. The most complete schema of the processes of stigmatization has four key components [18]: (i) labeling, in which personal characteristics are signaled or noted as conveying an important difference; (ii) stereotyping, where these differences are linked to undesirable characteristics; (iii) separating, where the categorical distinction is made between the mainstream/normal group and the labeled group; and (iv) status loss and discrimination, where the labeled group is devalued, rejected, and excluded. Interestingly, more recently the authors of this model have added a revision to include the emotional reactions of both those who are stigmatized and of the "stigmatizers", which may accompany each of these stages [19, 20].

Stigma can also be seen as an overarching term including three elements:

• problems of knowledge (ignorance or misinformation)

Community Mental Health: putting policy into practice globally, First Edition. Graham Thornicroft, Maya Semrau, Atalay Alem, Robert E. Drake, Hiroto Ito, Jair Mari, Peter McGeorge, and R. Thara. © 2011 John Wiley & Sons, Ltd. Published 2011 by John Wiley & Sons, Ltd.

- problems of attitudes (prejudice)
- problems of behavior (discrimination) [4, 18, 21].

Stigma may produce changes in feelings, attitudes, and behavior for both the person affected (lower self-esteem, poorer self-care, and social withdrawal) and their family members [14, 22–26]. Consistent findings have emerged from evaluating stigma in Africa [27], Asia [28], South America [29], Islamic countries of North Africa and the Near East [30], and Europe [12]. First, there are few countries, societies, or cultures in which people with mental illness are considered to have the same value as people who do not have mental illness, as shown for example by lower rates of financial investment in mental health services, which has been described as an aspect of *structural discrimination* (see below). Second, the quality of information that we have is relatively poor, with few comparative studies between countries or over time. Third, there are clear links between popular understandings of mental illness and whether people in mental distress seek help or feel able to disclose their problems [31].

The central experiences of shame (to oneself or to one's family) and blame (from others) are common, although they vary to some extent between cultures. Where comparisons with other conditions have been made, mental illnesses are usually more stigmatized, and indeed this has been called the "ultimate stigma" [7]. Finally, the behavioral consequences of stigma (rejection and avoidance) appear to be universal phenomena. Nevertheless, this literature says little about a core issue: how such processes affect the everyday lives of people with mental illness.

Studies on stigma and mental illness largely consist of attitude surveys, investigating what people would do in imaginary situations or what they think "most people" would do, for example, when faced with a neighbor or work colleague with mental illness. This work has emphasized what "normal" people say rather than the actual experiences of people with mental illness themselves. It also assumes that such statements (usually on knowledge, attitudes, or behavioural intentions) are linked with actual behavior, rather than assessing such behavior directly. In short, with some clear exceptions, this research has focused on hypothetical rather than real situations, shorn of emotions and feelings [32], divorced from context [33], indirectly rather than directly experienced, and without clear implications for how to intervene to reduce social rejection [34].

Recently a growing body of qualitative evidence has considered how mental health service users subjectively experience, describe, and cope with stigma. This has allowed an enhanced understanding of: the scope and dimensions of stigma; the personal consequences of stigma; mental health service users' views on anti-stigma campaign priorities; and the impact of stigma on the family—along with the development of related scales to measure stigma [35].

Understanding stigma is important because stigma can lead to low rates of help-seeking, lack of access to care, under-treatment, material poverty, and social marginalization [36, 37]. These effects can be the consequences of *experienced* (actual) discrimination (for example being unreasonably rejected in a job application) or of *anticipated* discrimination (for example not applying for a job because one expects to fail in any such application) [38, 39]. This distinction between experienced and anticipated discrimination is closely related to what has been described as the difference between "enacted" and "felt" stigma. "Enacted stigma" refers to events of negative discrimination, while "felt stigma" includes the experience of shame of having a condition and the fear of encountering "enacted stigma" [40], and is associated with lower self-esteem.

Ignorance: the problem of knowledge

There is an unprecedented volume of information in the public domain, but the level of accurate knowledge about mental illnesses (sometimes called "mental health literacy") is meager [41]. In a population survey in England, for example, most people (55%) believed that the statement "someone who cannot be held responsible for his or her own actions" describes a person who is mentally ill [42]. Most (63%) thought that fewer than 10% of the population would experience a mental illness at some time in their lives, a vast underestimation.

Prejudice: the problem of negative attitudes

The term "prejudice" is used to refer to the experience of disadvantage by many social groups, for example minority ethnic groups, yet it is employed rarely in relation to people with mental illness. The prejudice of a host majority to a minority group usually involves not just negative thoughts but also emotions such as anxiety, anger, resentment, hostility, distaste, or disgust. In fact, prejudice may more strongly predict discrimination than do stereotypes. Interestingly, there is almost nothing published about emotional reactions to people with mental illness apart from that which describes a fear of violence [43]. An example of such negative attitudes is the terms used by school students towards people with mental health problems; in one English study, among 250 such terms used, none were positive and 70% were negative [44, 45].

Discrimination: the problem of rejecting and avoidant behavior

Attitude and social-distance surveys (of unwillingness to have social contact) usually ask either students or members of the general public what they would do in imaginary situations or what they think "most people" would do, for example, when faced with a neighbor or work colleague with mental illness. Although such research is useful, as discussed above it has emphasized what "normal" people say rather than the experiences of people with mental illnesses themselves, and does not assess behavior and discrimination directly [46–49].

Structural discrimination

The concept of "structural discrimination" (sometimes called systemic discrimination) has been developed to mean "the policies of private and governmental institutions that intentionally restrict the opportunities of people with mental illness and policies of institutions that yield unintended consequences that hinder the options of people with mental illness" [33].

Corrigan et al. argue for further methodological and conceptual work to understand structural discrimination, and this will be of undoubted benefit [33]. Additionally, we argue that by publicizing structural discrimination in bold terms, and by relating macro-level analyses to the plight of individuals (in the way it was done in the wake of the Lawrence Inquiry), the stigma agenda may achieve similar prominence. People affected by stigma and mental illness are equal, if not greater in number, than those affected by institutional racism. We can learn important lessons from the successes of the UK race-relations struggle. Coupled with the impact of powerful domestic and European anti-discrimination laws and proven governmental goodwill and resources (e.g. the "See Me" anti-stigma campaign in Scotland [50]), the European anti-stigma movement has the ingredients to empower governments and institutions to tackle the problem of stigma and mental illness head on.

Global patterns of stigma and discrimination

Is it the case that stigma and discrimination vary between countries? The evidence here is stronger, but still frustratingly patchy [51]. Although studies on stigma and mental illness have been carried out in many countries, few have compared two or more places, or have included non-Western nations [52].

One study in Africa described attitudes to mentally ill people in rural sites in Ethiopia. Among almost 200 relatives of people with diagnoses of schizophrenia or mood disorders, 75% said that they had experienced stigma due to the presence of mental illness in the family, and a third (37%) wanted to conceal the fact that a relative was ill. Most family members (65%) said that praying was their preferred method of treating the condition [53]. Among the general population in Ethiopia, schizophrenia was judged to be the most severe problem, and talkativeness, aggression, and strange behavior were rated the most common symptoms of mental illness [27].

A survey was conducted in South Africa of over 600 members of the public on their knowledge of and attitudes towards people with mental illness [54–56]. Different vignettes, portraying depression, schizophrenia, panic disorder, and substance misuse, were presented to each person. Most thought that these conditions were related either to stress or to a lack of willpower, rather than seeing them as medical disorders [57]. Similar work in Turkey [58], and in Siberia and Mongolia [59], suggests that people in such countries may be more ready to make the individual responsible for his or her mental illness and less willing to grant the benefits of the sick role.

Although most of the published work on stigma is by authors in the USA and Canada [9, 60–62], there are also a few reports from elsewhere in the Americas and in the Caribbean [63]. In a review of studies from Argentina, Brazil, Dominica, Mexico, and Nicaragua, mainly from urban sites, a number of common themes emerged. The conditions most often rated as "mental illnesses" were psychotic disorders, especially schizophrenia. People with higher levels of education tended to have more favorable attitudes to people with mental illness. Alcoholism was considered to be the most common type of mental disorder. Most people thought that a health professional needs to be consulted by people with mental illnesses [29].

Some research has also been published concerning the question of stigma towards mentally ill people in Asian countries and cultures [64–66]. Within China [67], a large-scale survey was undertaken of over 600 people with a diagnosis of schizophrenia and over 900 family members [68]. Over half of the family members said that stigma had had an important effect on them and their family, and levels of stigmatization were higher in urban areas and for people who were more highly educated.

Within the field of stigma research it is clear that schizophrenia is the primary focus of interest. It is remarkable that there are almost no studies, for example, on bipolar disorder and stigma. A comparison of attitudes to schizophrenia was undertaken in England and Hong Kong. As predicted, the Chinese respondents expressed more negative attitudes and beliefs about schizophrenia, and preferred a more social model to explain its causation. In both countries, most participants, whatever their educational level, showed great ignorance about this condition [69]. This may be why most of the population in Hong Kong is very concerned about its mental health and holds rather negative views about mentally ill people [70]. Less favorable attitudes were common in those with less direct personal contact with people with mental illness (as in most Western studies), and in women (the opposite of what has been found in many Western reports) [71].

Although rather less research on stigma has been conducted in India, one study found that among relatives of people with schizophrenia in Chennai (Madras) in Southern India, their main concerns were: effects on marital prospects, fear of rejection by neighbors, and the need to hide the condition from others. Higher levels of stigma were reported by women and by younger people with the condition [72]. Women who have mental illness appear to be at a particular disadvantage in India. If they are divorced—sometimes related to concerns about heredity [73]—they often receive no financial support from their former husbands, and they and their families experience intense distress from the additional stigma of the separation or divorce [28].

Mental illnesses are seen in Japan as reflecting a loss of control, and so as not being subject to the force of willpower, leading to a sense of shame [74–76]. Although it is tempting to generalize about the degree of stigma in different countries, reality may not allow such simplifications. A comparison of attitudes to mentally ill people in Japan and Bali, for example, showed that views towards people with schizophrenia were less favorable in Japan, but that people with depression and obsessive–compulsive disorder were seen to be less acceptable in Bali [77].

Different countries do tend to share in common a high level of ignorance and misinformation about mental illnesses. A survey of teachers' opinions in Japan and Taiwan showed that relatively few could describe the main features of schizophrenia with any accuracy. The general profile of knowledge, beliefs, and attitudes was similar to that found in most Western countries, although the degree of social rejection was somewhat greater in Japan [78].

In 2002, the Japanese Society of Psychiatry and Neurology, at the request of a group of patients' families, reviewed the Japanese name for schizophrenia—"Seishin Bunretsu Byo" ("mind-split disease"). The group asked for a new name that was less stigmatizing and more accurate, and which represented the change in understanding of schizophrenia from a chronic incurable disease to one in which recovery was possible, and which acknowledged a biopsychosocial approach to the disease. Accordingly, the name was successfully changed to "Togo Shitcho Sho" ("integration disorder"), which within months was widely accepted amongst

Japanese mental health professionals, who indicated that it became easier to explain the diagnosis to patients, establish a therapeutic relationship, improve concordance, and reduce stigma. [79] Moreover, the change in name has led to indications from service users and their families that they feel able to discuss the illness more openly as a result.

What is known from the English-language literature of stigma in Islamic communities? Despite earlier indications that the intensity of stigma may be relatively low here [66], detailed studies indicate that, on balance, it is no less than we have seen described elsewhere [80–83]. A study of family members in Morocco found that 76% had no knowledge about the condition, and many considered it chronic (80%), handicapping (48%), incurable (39%), or linked with sorcery (25%). Most said that they had "hard lives" because of the diagnosis [25]. Turning to religious authority figures is reported to be common in some Muslim countries [30,84]. Some studies have found that direct personal contact is not associated with more favorable attitudes to people with mental illness [85,86], especially where behavior is seen to threaten the social fabric of the community [58,87].

A recent global survey used the Discrimination and Stigma Scale (DISC) in a cross-sectional survey in 27 countries, using language-equivalent versions of the instrument in face-to-face interviews between research staff and 732 participants with a clinical diagnosis of schizophrenia [39]. The most frequently occurring areas of negative experienced discrimination were: making or keeping friends (47%), discrimination by family members (43%), keeping a job (29%), finding a job (29%), and intimate or sexual relationships (29%) (see Figure 7.1). Positive experienced discrimination was rare. Anticipated discrimination was common for: applying for work, training, or education (64%) and looking for a close relationship (55%); 72% felt the need to conceal the diagnosis (see Figure 7.2). Anticipated discrimination occurred more often than experienced discrimination. This study suggests that rates of experienced discrimination are relatively high and consistent across countries. For two of the most important domains (work and personal relationships), anticipated discrimination occurs in the absence of experienced discrimination in over a third of participants. This has important implications: disability discrimination laws may not be effective without also developing interventions to reduce anticipated discrimination, for example by enhancing the self-esteem of people with mental illness, so that they will be more likely to apply for jobs.

Prejudice and discrimination by the public against people with mental illness are therefore common, deeply socially damaging, and part of more widespread stigmatization. Stigma against people with mental illness can contribute to negative outcomes, as well as perpetuating self-stigmatization and contributing to low self-esteem.

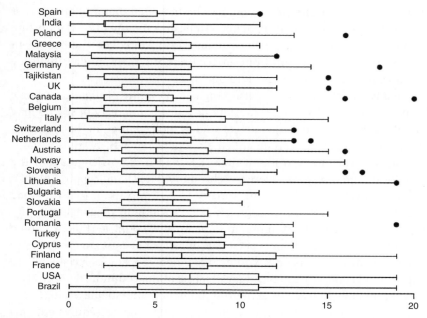

Figure 7.1 Negative experienced discrimination by country in the INDIGO Study (from Thornicroft et al. 2009 [39]). The axis shows the range from least (0) to most (32) domains of discrimination. Data show medians, inter-quartile ranges, total ranges, and outliers.

Yet it remains the case that addressing public "knowledge" and "attitudes", as discussed above, does not necessarily lead to a change in "behavior" and "discrimination". This remains an elusive goal and further work is needed to understand the complex relationships between these

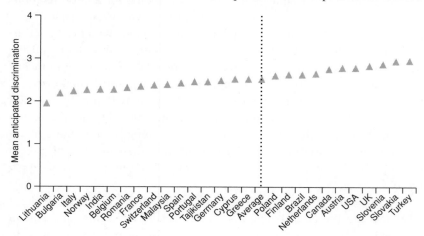

Figure 7.2 Mean anticipated discrimination by country in the INDIGO study (from Thornicroft et al. 2009 [39]).
Key: possible range 0–4.

elements of stigma, and to identify and develop evidence-based tools and interventions with which to tackle discrimination.

Community awareness about mental illnesses

A common barrier in identifying and treating mental disorders worldwide is the lack of awareness about them within communities, with stigma towards, and discrimination against, people with mental health problems being widespread. This is important, because effective awareness-raising campaigns can result in increased presentation of persons with mental illness to primary health care [88].

Three main strategies have been used to reduce public stigma and discrimination: protest, education, and social contact [89]. Protest, by stigmatized individuals or members of the public who support them, is often applied against stigmatizing public statements, such as media reports and advertisements. Many protest interventions, for instance against stigmatizing advertisements or soap operas, have successfully suppressed negative public statements, and for this purpose they are clearly very useful [90]. However, it has been argued that protest is not effective for improving attitudes toward people with mental illness [89].

Education interventions aim to diminish stigma by replacing myths and negative stereotypes with facts, and have reduced stigmatizing attitudes among members of the public. However, research on educational campaigns suggests that behavior changes are often not evaluated.

The third strategy is personal social contact with persons with mental illness [22]. For example, in a number of interventions in secondary schools, or with the police, education and personal social contact have been combined [91, 92]. Social contact appears to be the more efficacious part of the intervention. Factors that create an advantageous environment for interpersonal contact and stigma reduction may include equal status among participants, a cooperative interaction, and institutional support for the contact initiative [93].

For both education and contact, the content of programs against stigma and discrimination matters. Biogenetic models of mental illness are often highlighted because viewing mental illness as a biological, mainly inherited problem may reduce shame and blame associated with it. Evidence supports this optimistic expectation (i.e. that a biogenetic causal model of mental illness will reduce stigma) in terms of reduced blame. However, focusing on biogenetic factors may increase the perception that people with mental illness are fundamentally different, and thus biogenetic interpretations have been associated with increased social distance [94]. Therefore, a message of mental illness as being "genetic" or "neurological" may be overly simplistic and unhelpful for reducing stigma. Indeed, in many low- and middle-income countries, conveying a message emphasizing the heritable nature of mental illness fuels stigma, for instance making marriage more difficult.

With a growing awareness about such stigma, a number of recent initiatives have been launched in the UK aiming to improve public attitudes. The Royal College of Psychiatrists' "Changing Minds" campaign in England ran between 1998 and 2003. It advertised Web sites, showed campaign videos in cinemas, distributed leaflets to the general public and health care professionals, and created reading material for young people for use in the curriculum [41, 96, 97].

The Scottish Executive's "See Me" campaign (2002–present) has a higher profile, is better funded, and is more extensive. It aims to deliver specific messages to the Scottish population by using all forms of media, as well as cinema advertising, outdoor posters, and supporting leaflets in GP surgeries, libraries, prisons, schools, and youth groups. It also has a detailed Web site containing interactive resources, and its impact is regularly monitored and its progress reported in the public domain [98]. The investment of public funds in government campaigns is an important step, and evidence suggesting that "See Me" may have had a positive effect on attitudes in Scotland relative to England is encouraging [98–99].

In a campaign in Australia to increase knowledge about depression and its treatment, some states and territories received an intensive, coordinated program, while others did not. In the former, people more often recognized the features of depression, and were more likely to support help-seeking for depression or to accept treatment with counseling and medication [100].

A new campaign is now starting in England, entitled "Time to Change", aiming to fundamentally reduce stigma and discrimination [46, 48, 95]. This large, multifaceted national campaign combines mass-media advertising and local initiatives. The latter try to facilitate social contact between members of the general public and mental health service users, as well as target specific groups such as medical students and teachers. The program is evaluated by public surveys assessing knowledge, attitudes, and behavior, and by measuring the amount of experienced discrimination reported by people with mental illness. Similar initiatives in other countries, such as "Like Minds, Like Mine" in New Zealand [101] or the World Psychiatric Association's anti-stigma initiative [102], and other programs in Japan, Brazil, Egypt and Nigeria [88], have reported positive outcomes.

In sum, there is evidence for the effectiveness of measures against stigma and against discrimination [39]. On a more cautious note, individual discrimination, structural discrimination, and self-stigma lead to innumerable mechanisms of stigmatization. If one mechanism of discrimination is blocked or diminished through successful initiatives, other ways to discriminate may emerge [103, 104]. Therefore, to substantially reduce discrimination, the stigmatizing attitudes and behaviors of influential stakeholders need to change fundamentally.

Key points in this chapter

- Stigma and discrimination appear to be universal phenomena.
- A lack of awareness within communities about mental disorders, as well as stigma towards and discrimination against people with mental health problems, are common across countries. This may often act as a barrier in identifying and treating mental disorders.
- Effective awareness-raising campaigns can result in increased presentation of persons with mental illness to primary health care.
- Strategies used to reduce public stigma and discrimination include protest, education, and social contact. Whilst it is unclear whether protest is effective in improving the public's attitudes towards people with mental health problems, education and social contact have been found to improve people's attitudes and reduce stigma. However, the content of such programs is an important factor in determining whether attitudes and behaviors change for the better.

References

[1] Gilman SL. Seeing the Insane. Wiley: New York; 1982.
[2] Gilman SL. Difference and Pathology: Stereotypes of Sexuality, Race and Madness. Ithaca: Cornell University Press; 1985.
[3] Goffman I. Stigma: Notes on the Management of Spoiled Identity. Harmondsworth, Middlesex: Penguin Books; 1963.
[4] Scambler G. Stigma and disease: changing paradigms. Lancet 1998;352(9133): 1054–5.
[5] Hinshaw SP, Cicchetti D. Stigma and mental disorder: conceptions of illness, public attitudes, personal disclosure, and social policy. Dev Psychopathol 2000;12(4):555–98.
[6] Mason T. Stigma and Social Exclusion in Healthcare. London: Routledge; 2001.
[7] Falk G. Stigma: How We Treat Outsiders. New York: Prometheus Books; 2001.
[8] Heatherton TF, Kleck RE, Hebl MR, Hull JG. The Social Psychology of Stigma. New York: Guilford Press; 2003.
[9] Corrigan P. On the Stigma of Mental Illness. Washington, DC: American Psychological Association; 2005.
[10] Wahl OF. Telling is a Risky Business: Mental Health Consumers Confront Stigma. New Jersey: Rutgers University Press; 1999.
[11] Pickenhagen A, Sartorius N. The WPA Global Programme to Reduce Stigma and Discrimination because of Schizophrenia. Geneva: WPA; 2002.

[12] Sartorius N, Schulze H. Reducing the Stigma of Mental Illness: A Report from a Global Association. Cambridge: Cambridge University Press; 2005.

[13] Hayward P, Bright JA. Stigma and mental illness: A review and critique. Journal of Mental Health 1997;6(4):345–54.

[14] Link BG, Cullen FT, Struening EL, Shrout PE, Dohrenwend BP. A modified labeling theory approach in the area of mental disorders: An empirical assessment. American Sociological Review 1989;54:100–23.

[15] Link BG, Struening EL, Rahav M, Phelan JC, Nuttbrock L. On stigma and its consequences: evidence from a longitudinal study of men with dual diagnoses of mental illness and substance abuse. J Health Soc Behav 1997;38(2):177–90.

[16] Link BG, Phelan JC, Bresnahan M, Stueve A, Pescosolido BA. Public conceptions of mental illness: labels, causes, dangerousness, and social distance. Am J Public Health 1999;89(9):1328–33.

[17] Smith M. Stigma. Advances in Psychiatric Treatment 2002;8:317–25.

[18] Link BG, Phelan JC. Conceptualizing stigma. Annual Review of Sociology 2001;27:363–85.

[19] Link BG, Yang LH, Phelan JC, Collins PY. Measuring mental illness stigma. Schizophr Bull 2004;30(3):511–41.

[20] Jones E, Farina A, Hastorf A, Markus H, Milller D, Scott R. Social Stigma: The Psychology of Marked to Relationships. New York: W.H. Freeman & Co.; 1984.

[21] Hinshaw S. The Mark of Shame. Oxford: Oxford University Press; 2007.

[22] Thornicroft G. Shunned: Discrimination against People with Mental Illness. Oxford: Oxford University Press; 2006.

[23] Littlewood R, Jadhav S, Ryder AG. A cross-national study of the stigmatization of severe psychiatric illness: historical review, methodological considerations and development of the questionnaire. Transcult Psychiatry 2007;44(2):171–202.

[24] Weiss MG, Jadhav S, Raguram R, Vaunatsou P, Littlewood L. Psychiatric stigma across cultures: local validation in Bangalore and London. Anthropology & Medicine 2001;8:71–87.

[25] Kadri N, Manoudi F, Berrada S, Moussaoui D. Stigma impact on Moroccan families of patients with schizophrenia. Can J Psychiatry 2004;49(9):625–9.

[26] Ritsher JB, Phelan JC. Internalized stigma predicts erosion of morale among psychiatric outpatients. Psychiatry Res 2004;129(3):257–65.

[27] Alem A, Jacobsson L, Araya M, Kebede D, Kullgren G. How are mental disorders seen and where is help sought in a rural Ethiopian community? A key informant study in Butajira, Ethiopia. Acta Psychiatr Scand Suppl 1999;397:40–7.

[28] Thara R, Kamath S, Kumar S. Women with schizophrenia and broken marriages: Doubly disadvantaged? Part II. Family perspective. Int J Soc Psychiatry 2003;49(3):233–40.

[29] de Toledo Piza PE, Blay SL. Community perception of mental disorders: a systematic review of Latin American and Caribbean studies. Soc Psychiatry Psychiatr Epidemiol 2004;39(12):955–61.

[30] Al-Krenawi A, Graham JR, Dean YZ, Eltaiba N. Cross-national study of attitudes towards seeking professional help: Jordan, United Arab Emirates (UAE) and Arabs in Israel. Int J Soc Psychiatry 2004;50(2):102–14.

[31] Littlewood R. Cultural variation in the stigmatisation of mental illness. Lancet 1998;352(9133):1056–7.

[32] Crocker J, Major B., Steele C. Social Stigma. In: Gilbert D, Fiske ST, Lindzey G, editors. The Handbook of Social Psychology. 4th ed. Boston: McGraw-Hill; 1998. pp. 504–33.

[33] Corrigan PW, Markowitz FE, Watson AC. Structural levels of mental illness stigma and discrimination. Schizophr Bull 2004;30(3):481–91.

[34] Rose D. Users' Voices: The Perspectives of Mental Health Service Users on Community and Hospital Care. London: The Sainsbury Centre; 2001.

[35] King M, Dinos S, Shaw J, Watson R, Stevens S, Passetti F, et al. The Stigma Scale: Development of a standardised measure of the stigma of mental illness. Br J Psychiatry 2007;190(3):248–54.

[36] Thornicroft G. Most people with mental illness are not treated. Lancet 2007;370(9590):807–8.

[37] Thornicroft G. Stigma and discrimination limit access to mental health care. Epidemiol Psichiatr Soc 2008;17(1):14–19.

[38] Rusch N, Angermeyer MC, Corrigan PW. [The stigma of mental illness: concepts, forms, and consequences.] Psychiatr Prax 2005;32(5):221–32.

[39] Thornicroft G, Brohan E, Rose D, Sartorius N, Leese M, INDIGO Study Group. Global pattern of experienced and anticipated discrimination against people with schizophrenia: A cross-sectional survey. Lancet 2009;373:408–15.

[40] Jacoby A. Felt versus enacted stigma: A concept revisited—Evidence from a study of people with epilepsy in remission. Soc Sci Med 1994;38(2):269–74.

[41] Crisp A, Gelder MG, Goddard E, Meltzer H. Stigmatization of people with mental illnesses: A follow-up study within the Changing Minds campaign of the Royal College of Psychiatrists. World Psychiatry 2005;4:106–13.

[42] Department of Health. Attitudes to Mental Illness 2003 Report. London: Department of Health; 2003.

[43] Graves RE, Cassisi JE, Penn DL. Psychophysiological evaluation of stigma towards schizophrenia. Schizophr Res 2005;76(2–3):317–27.

[44] Rose D, Thornicroft G, Pinfold V, Kassam A. 250 labels used to stigmatise people with mental illness. BMC Health Serv Res 2007;7:97.

[45] Pinfold V, Toulmin H, Thornicroft G, Huxley P, Farmer P, Graham T. Reducing psychiatric stigma and discrimination: evaluation of educational interventions in UK secondary schools. British Journal of Psychiatry 2003;182:342–6.

[46] Hamilton S, Pinfold V, Rose D, Henderson C, Lewis-Holmes E, Flach C, et al. The effect of disclosure of mental illness by interviewers on reports of discrimination experienced by service users: A randomized study. Int Rev Psychiatry 2011;23(1):47–54.

[47] Wheat K, Brohan E, Henderson C, Thornicroft G. Mental illness and the workplace: Conceal or reveal? J R Soc Med 2010;103(3):83–6.

[48] Clement S, Jarrett M, Henderson C, Thornicroft G. Messages to use in population-level campaigns to reduce mental health-related stigma: Consensus development study. Epidemiol Psichiatr Soc 2010;19(1):72–9.

[49] Evans-Lacko S, Little K, Meltzer H, Rose D, Rhydderch D, Henderson C, et al. Development and psychometric properties of the Mental Health Knowledge Schedule. Can J Psychiatry 2010;55(7):440–8.

[50] See Me. See Me So Far: A review of the first four years of the Scottish Anti Stigma Campaign. Edinburgh: Scottish Executive; 2007.

[51] Littlewood R. Cultural and national aspects of stigmatisation. In: Crisp AH, editor. Every Family in the Land. London: Royal Society of Medicine; 2004. pp. 14–17.

[52] Fabrega H, Jr. The culture and history of psychiatric stigma in early modern and modern Western societies: A review of recent literature. Compr Psychiatry 1991;32(2):97–119.

[53] Shibre T, Negash A, Kullgren G, Kebede D, Alem A, Fekadu A, et al. Perception of stigma among family members of individuals with schizophrenia and major affective disorders in rural Ethiopia. Soc Psychiatry Psychiatr Epidemiol 2001;36(6):299–303.

[54] Stein DJ, Wessels C, Van Kradenberg J, Emsley RA. The Mental Health Information Centre of South Africa: A report of the first 500 calls. Cent Afr J Med 1997;43(9):244–6.

[55] Minde M. History of mental health services in South Africa. Part XIII. The National Council for Mental Health. S Afr Med J 1976;50(3F):1452–6.

[56] Hugo CJ, Boshoff DE, Traut A, Zungu-Dirwayi N, Stein DJ. Community attitudes toward and knowledge of mental illness in South Africa. Soc Psychiatry Psychiatr Epidemiol 2003;38(12):715–19.

[57] Cheetham WS, Cheetham RJ. Concepts of mental illness amongst the rural Xhosa people in South Africa. Aust N Z J Psychiatry 1976;10(1):39–45.

[58] Ozmen E, Ogel K, Aker T, Sagduyu A, Tamar D, Boratav C. Public attitudes to depression in urban Turkey: the influence of perceptions and causal attributions on social distance towards individuals suffering from depression. Soc Psychiatry Psychiatr Epidemiol 2004;39(12):1010–16.

[59] Dietrich S, Beck M, Bujantugs B, Kenzine D, Matschinger H, Angermeyer MC. The relationship between public causal beliefs and social distance toward mentally ill people. Aust N Z J Psychiatry 2004;38(5):348–54.

[60] Link BG, Yang LH, Phelan JC, Collins PY. Measuring mental illness stigma. Schizophr Bull 2004;30(3):511–41.

[61] Estroff SE, Penn DL, Toporek JR. From stigma to discrimination: An analysis of community efforts to reduce the negative consequences of having a psychiatric disorder and label. Schizophr Bull 2004;30(3):493–509.

[62] Corrigan P, Thompson V, Lambert D, Sangster Y, Noel JG, Campbell J. Perceptions of discrimination among persons with serious mental illness. Psychiatr Serv 2003;54(8):1105–10.

[63] Villares C, Sartorius N. Challenging the stigma of schizophrenia. Rev Bras Psiquiatr 2003;25:1–2.

[64] Ng CH. The stigma of mental illness in Asian cultures. Aust N Z J Psychiatry 1997;31(3):382–90.

[65] Leong FT, Lau AS. Barriers to providing effective mental health services to Asian Americans. Ment Health Serv Res 2001 Dec;3(4):201–14.

[66] Fabrega H, Jr. Psychiatric stigma in non-Western societies. Compr Psychiatry 1991;32(6):534–51.

[67] Kleinman A, Mechanic D. Some observations of mental illness and its treatment in the People's Republic of China. J Nerv Ment Dis 1979;167(5):267–74.

[68] Phillips MR, Pearson V, Li F, Xu M, Yang L. Stigma and expressed emotion: A study of people with schizophrenia and their family members in China. Br J Psychiatry 2002;181:488–93.

[69] Furnham A, Chan E. Lay theories of schizophrenia: A cross-cultural comparison of British and Hong Kong Chinese attitudes, attributions and beliefs. Soc Psychiatry Psychiatr Epidemiol 2004;39(7):543–52.

[70] Chou KL, Mak KY, Chung PK, Ho K. Attitudes towards mental patients in Hong Kong. Int J Soc Psychiatry 1996;42(3):213–19.

[71] Chung KF, Chen EY, Liu CS. University students' attitudes towards mental patients and psychiatric treatment. Int J Soc Psychiatry 2001;47(2):63–72.

[72] Thara R, Srinivasan TN. How stigmatising is schizophrenia in India? Int J Soc Psychiatry 2000;46(2):135–41.

[73] Raguram R, Raghu TM, Vounatsou P, Weiss MG. Schizophrenia and the cultural epidemiology of stigma in Bangalore, India. J Nerv Ment Dis 2004;192(11): 734–44.

[74] Desapriya EB, Nobutada I. Stigma of mental illness in Japan. Lancet 2002; 359(9320):1866.

[75] Hasui C, Sakamoto S, Suguira B, Kitamura T. Stigmatization of mental illness in Japan: Images and frequency of encounters with diagnostic categories of mental illness among medical and non-medical university students. Journal of Psychiatry & Law 2000;28(Summer):253–66.

[76] Sugiura T, Sakamoto S, Kijima N, Kitamura F, Kitamura T. Stigmatizing perception of mental illness by Japanese students: Comparison of different psychiatric disorders. J Nerv Ment Dis 2000;188(4):239–42.

[77] Kurihara T, Kato M, Sakamoto S, Reverger R, Kitamura T. Public attitudes towards the mentally ill: A cross-cultural study between Bali and Tokyo. Psychiatry Clin Neurosci 2000;54(5):547–52.

[78] Kurumatani T, Ukawa K, Kawaguchi Y, Miyata S, Suzuki M, Ide H, et al. Teachers' knowledge, beliefs and attitudes concerning schizophrenia- a cross-cultural approach in Japan and Taiwan. Soc Psychiatry Psychiatr Epidemiol 2004;39(5):402–9.

[79] Sato M. Renaming schizophrenia: A Japanese perspective. World Psychiatry 2009;5(1):53–5.

[80] Karim S, Saeed K, Rana MH, Mubbashar MH, Jenkins R. Pakistan mental health country profile. Int Rev Psychiatry 2004;16(1–2):83–92.

[81] Al-Krenawi A, Graham JR, Kandah J. Gendered utilization differences of mental health services in Jordan. Community Ment Health J 2000;36(5):501–11.

[82] Al-Krenawi A, Graham JR, Ophir M, Kandah J. Ethnic and gender differences in mental health utilization: the case of Muslim Jordanian and Moroccan Jewish Israeli out-patient psychiatric patients. Int J Soc Psychiatry 2001;47(3):42–54.

[83] Cinnirella M, Loewenthal KM. Religious and ethnic group influences on beliefs about mental illness: A qualitative interview study. Br J Med Psychol 1999;72(4):505–24.

[84] Loewenthal KM, Cinnirella M, Evdoka G, Murphy P. Faith conquers all? Beliefs about the role of religious factors in coping with depression among different cultural-religious groups in the UK. Br J Med Psychol 2001 Sep;74(3):293–303.

[85] Arkar H, Eker D. Influence of having a hospitalized mentally ill member in the family on attitudes toward mental patients in Turkey. Soc Psychiatry Psychiatr Epidemiol 1992;27(3):151–5.

[86] Arkar H, Eker D. Effect of psychiatric labels on attitudes toward mental illness in a Turkish sample. Int J Soc Psychiatry 1994;40(3):205–13.

[87] Coker EM. Selfhood and social distance: toward a cultural understanding of psychiatric stigma in Egypt. Soc Sci Med 2005;61(5):920–30.

[88] Eaton J, Agomoh AO. Developing mental health services in Nigeria: the impact of a community-based mental health awareness programme. Social Psychiatry and Psychiatric Epidemiology 2008; 43(7):552–8.

[89] Corrigan PW, Penn DL. Lessons from social psychology on discrediting psychiatric stigma. American Psychologist 1999;54:765–76.

[90] Wahl OF. Media madness: Public images of mental illness. New Brunswick: Rutgers University Press; 1995.

[91] Pinfold V, Huxley P, Thornicroft G, Farmer P, Toulmin H, Graham T. Reducing psychiatric stigma and discrimination–evaluating an educational intervention with the police force in England. Social Psychiatry and Psychiatric Epidemiology 2003;38:337–44.

[92] Pinfold V, Toulmin H, Thornicroft G, Huxley P, Farmer P, Graham T. Reducing psychiatric stigma and discrimination: evaluation of educational interventions in UK secondary schools. British Journal of Psychiatry 2003;182:342–6.

[93] Pinfold V, Thornicroft G, Huxley P, Farmer P. Active ingredients in anti-stigma programmes in mental health. International Review of Psychiatry 2005;17(2):123–31.

[94] Phelan JC, Yang LH, Cruz-Rojas R. Effects of attributing serious mental illnesses to genetic causes on orientations to treatment. Psychiatric Services 2006;57:382–7.

[95] Henderson C, Thornicroft G. Stigma and discrimination in mental illness: Time to change. Lancet 2009;373:1928–30.

[96] Crisp AH, Cowan L, Hart D. The college's anti-stigma campaign 1998–2003. Psychiatr Bull 2004;28:133–6.

[97] Crisp A. Every Family in the Land: Understanding Prejudice and Discrimination against People with Mental Illness. London: Royal Society of Medicine Press; 2004.

[98] Dunion L, Gordon L. Tackling the attitude problem. The achievements to date of Scotland's "See Me" anti-stigma campaign. Ment Health Today 2005(March); 22–5.

[99] Mehta N, Kassam A, Leese M, Butler G, Thornicroft G. Public attitudes towards people with mental illness in England and Scotland, 1994–2003. British Journal of Psychiatry 2009;194:278–84.

[100] Jorm AF, Christensen H, Griffiths KM. The impact of beyondblue: the national depression initiative on the Australian public's recognition of depression and beliefs about treatments. Aust N Z J Psychiatry 2005;39(4):248–54.

[101] Vaughan G, Hansen C. "Like Minds, Like Mine": A New Zealand project to counter the stigma and discrimination associated with mental illness. Australasian Psychiatry 2004;12:113–17.

[102] Sartorius N, Schulze H. Reducing the stigma of mental illness: A report from a Global Programme of the World Psychiatric Association. Cambridge: Cambridge University Press; 2005.

[103] Link BG, Phelan JC. Conceptualizing stigma. Annual Review of Sociology 2001;27:363–85.

[104] Corrigan PW, Larson JE, Rüsch N. Self-stigma and the "why try" effect: Impact on life goals and evidence-based practices. World Psychiatry 2009;8:75–81.

CHAPTER 8

Developing a consensus for engagement

Stakeholders in mental health care

The collaborative engagement of a wide variety of supportive stakeholders is critical to the successful implementation of community-oriented mental health care. This array of interest groups in mental health may include: politicians, provider organizations' executive and non-executive board members, health care managers, clinicians, key members of the community including NGO providers, service users and their families, and traditional and religious healers [1]. To involve them in the imperative for change will require different strategies, sometimes using a change-management team. Overall, having clear reasons for the shift to community-oriented care is essential, along with specific objectives. However, the work undertaken for this book has shown that there is still some way to go in developing a consensus across many stakeholders, in part possibly because there is still disagreement about what community mental health care actually entails.

Case study: stakeholder engagement in sub-Saharan Arica

In the WHO Mental Health Atlas [2], there was evidence of diverse interpretations of the meaning of community care across African countries [3–6], including: psychiatric nurses working with traditional healers and religious leaders, countrywide mental health promotion, the ability of primary care workers to diagnose and treat mental disorders, home visits by psychiatric nurses to recently discharged patients, follow-up of discharged patients, traditional medicine only, private medical practice, NGOs, healing centers, private clinics and traditional healers, outreach services and community care teams, and agricultural psychiatric rehabilitation services [2].

Community Mental Health: putting policy into practice globally, First Edition. Graham Thornicroft, Maya Semrau, Atalay Alem, Robert E. Drake, Hiroto Ito, Jair Mari, Peter McGeorge, and R. Thara. © 2011 John Wiley & Sons, Ltd. Published 2011 by John Wiley & Sons, Ltd.

In the survey of regional experts across Africa (see Chapter 1 for details), respondents from Nigeria, Sudan, and Tanzania expressed agreement with our working definition of community mental health care:

> Mental health services provided outside of hospital-based (general and psychiatric, inpatient and outpatient) services includes mental health care provision in primary care. It also includes specialist community mental health services.

However, as with the WHO Mental Health Atlas [2], a diversity of conceptualizations of community care was apparent. For many respondents, community mental health care on the ground did not involve specialist mental health workers (Kenya, Niger, and Liberia), and was conceptualized as the provision of mental health care by primary health care workers. The need to "move beyond the clinic" was emphasized by a Nigerian NGO, with community care including rehabilitation and due attention to human rights, empowerment, livelihood schemes, and involvement in education.

Respondents from Uganda noted the importance of traditional healers and community volunteers in the delivery of community-based mental health care. In Zimbabwe, community mental health care was defined as *"Where services in the community have been empowered to the community"*. Respondents from South Africa were more likely to define community mental health care in terms of a multidisciplinary team of specialist mental health workers providing clinical care and outreach services, integrated with primary health care services and interfacing with day centers, supported living units, residential care, and rehabilitation services [7–9].

Developing consensus for change therefore requires a great deal of preparatory investment of time spent meeting and communicating with people, to ensure that all stakeholders understand the processes involved. This includes both those groups necessary to allow proposals to proceed, and those groups who have the power to veto or stop the service developments. The main means of communication need to include written material and opportunities to meet with stakeholder groups. Politicians and administrators will require a compelling business case, usually very briefly expressed, and enhanced if economic data are available. However, others will need summaries of plans, slide presentations, and the opportunity to meet and work through proposals and concerns. Emails and Web site information and surveys are now valuable supplements to the process. The emphasis must be on a willingness to communicate in good faith and to do so openly and honestly doing "what it takes" to convince people of the benefits of the change process.

It is important to bear in mind that in some cases prejudice and self-interest will have to be confronted. It is helpful, at the beginning of the process, to identify both those who are likely to support change, and those who are likely to oppose it. A willingness to listen to concerns and to find ways of incorporating them, if possible, into the planning and implementation process is essential because, when such an attitude is communicated, there is an opportunity for people to feel included in the process. That done, boldness and firmness will communicate to remaining detractors the seriousness of the intent to implement change; it will also encourage supporters to believe that their aspirations for better mental health care will be realized, and thus embolden them in turn.

Engaging stakeholders requires both formal and informal opportunities to meet, receive advice, and work through issues. The establishment of broadly based reference groups early on in the change process is a key formal mechanism to achieving this [10, 11]. These should include all the key stakeholders, in particular service users, families, clinicians, and service providers, with the latter being essential to facilitate integrated systems of care further on in the process. While it is important to structure the overall process with formal meetings and communications, it is also important to be willing to convene informal meetings upon request to "troubleshoot" situations of concern. The consultation process should result in an amalgam of "bottom-up" and "top-down" contributions to the change process. Reports on progress are an essential way of maintaining trust and building excitement for the process of successful implementation.

It is also important to bear in mind that good mental health services have established processes for ensuring that the voices of service users, their families, and community providers are heard on an ongoing basis. Service users' views are important since their perception of their needs may vary from that of clinicians [12, 13] Moreover, outcome data rated by service users may be more important than those rated by staff [14]. A study in Italy found that service user-rated unmet needs predicted quality of life, whilst staff-rated unmet needs were not associated with service users' quality of life [15]. Furthermore, service users of a community mental health team reported a high desire for information and a degree of shared decision-making [16]. Similarly, service users of a crisis resolution team in Norway valued the greater sense of control that the service provided, as well as improved opportunities for participation in management decisions, and the sense of being seen and listened to [17].

In the USA approximately half of all people with severe and persistent mental illnesses receive no mental health services, often because they have rejected the available services [18]. Many others who have received mental health services have expressed dissatisfaction with the services. Users of the mental health system (variously called patients, clients, users, consumers, or survivors) have lodged strong objections to the existing mental health system. They have also argued that professionals' goal of stabilization does not correspond to their aspirations for recovery [19, 20], a concept defined on a per-individual basis, but which typically encompasses opportunities for education, work, friendship, independent living, and community participation [21]. They have also argued for meaningful roles in making decisions and in delivering mental health care, and for the elimination of coercion in the contexts of hospitalization, prescribing of medications, and outpatient treatment.

The aim is therefore not simply to achieve discontinuous change, but to promote an ongoing quality improvement in which consumers of mental health services know they have a major stake. Without such effective and united consortia, policy makers may find it easy to disregard the different demands of a fragmented mental health sector, and instead respond positively to health domains (e.g. HIV/AIDS) which demonstrate the self-discipline of a united approach with a small number of fully agreed priorities. In the long run it is the views of people with mental illness and their carers which offer the most reliable guide when deciding what to do next to improve mental health care [22].

Key points in this chapter

- The collaborative engagement of a wide range of stakeholders is essential to the successful implementation of community-oriented mental health care. This may include politicians, board members, health managers, clinicians, key members of the community including NGO providers, service users and their families, and traditional and religious healers.
- Having clear reasons and objectives for the shift to community-oriented care is essential. Messages should be concise, backed by evidence, and consistent.
- Developing consensus for change needs to involve meeting and communicating with all stakeholders. It should involve both formal and informal opportunities to meet, receive advice, and work through issues. The voices of service users, their families, and community providers should be heard on an ongoing basis.
- At times prejudice and self-interest may have to be confronted.

References

[1] Thornicroft G, Tansella M. Better Mental Health Care. Cambridge: Cambridge University Press; 2009.
[2] World Health Organization. Mental Health Atlas, revised edition. 2005.

[3] Kleintjes S, Lund C, Flisher AJ. A situational analysis of child and adolescent mental health services in Ghana, Uganda, South Africa and Zambia. Afr J Psychiatry (Johannesbg) 2010;13(2):132–9.

[4] Ssebunnya J, Kigozi F, Lund C, Kizza D, Okello E. Stakeholder perceptions of mental health stigma and poverty in Uganda. BMC Int Health Hum Rights 2009;9:5.

[5] Mwape L, Sikwese A, Kapungwe A, Mwanza J, Flisher A, Lund C, et al. Integrating mental health into primary health care in Zambia: A care provider's perspective. Int J Ment Health Syst 2010;4:21.

[6] Lund C. Mental health in Africa: Findings from the Mental Health and Poverty Project. Int Rev Psychiatry 2010;22(6):547–9.

[7] Petersen I, Bhana A, Campbell-Hall V, Mjadu S, Lund C, Kleintjies S, et al. Planning for district mental health services in South Africa: A situational analysis of a rural district site. Health Policy Plan 2009;24(2):140–50.

[8] Lund C, Flisher AJ. A model for community mental health services in South Africa. Trop Med Int Health 2009;14(9):1040–7.

[9] Lund C, Kleintjes S, Kakuma R, Flisher AJ. Public sector mental health systems in South Africa: Inter-provincial comparisons and policy implications. Soc Psychiatry Psychiatr Epidemiol 2010;45(3):393–404.

[10] Thornicroft G, Tansella M, Law A. Steps, challenges and lessons in developing community mental health care. World Psychiatry 2008;7(2):87–92.

[11] Thornicroft G, Alem A, Atunes dos Santos R, Barley E, Drake R, Gregorio F, et al. WPA guidance on steps, obstacles and mistakes to avoid in the implementation of community mental health care. World Psychiatry 2010;9:67–77.

[12] Slade M. Assessing the needs of the severely mentally ill: Cultural and professional differences. Int J Soc Psychiatry 1996;42(1):1–9.

[13] Slade M, Leese M, Cahill S, Thornicroft G, Kuipers E. Patient-rated mental health needs and quality of life improvement. Br J Psychiatry 2005;187:256–61.

[14] Thornicroft G, Tansella M. Growing recognition of the importance of service user involvement in mental health service planning and evaluation. Epidemiologia e Psichiatria Sociale 2005;14(1):1–3.

[15] Slade M, Leese M, Ruggeri M, Kuipers E, Tansella M, Thornicroft G. Does meeting needs improve quality of life? Psychotherapy & Psychosomatics 2004;73(3):183–9.

[16] Hill SA, Laugharne R. Decision making and information seeking preferences among psychiatric patients. Journal of Mental Health 2006;15(1):75–84.

[17] Karlsson B, Borg M, Kim HS. From good intentions to real life: Introducing crisis resolution teams in Norway. Nurs Inq 2008;15(3):206–15.

[18] Mojtabai R, Fochtmann L, Chang S, Kotov R, Craig TJ, Bromet E. Unmet need for mental health care in schizophrenia: An overview of literature and new data from a first-admission study. Schizophrenia Bulletin 2009;35(4):679–95.

[19] Deegan P. Recovery: The lived experience of rehabilitation. Psychosocial Rehabilitation 1988;11:11–9.

[20] Slade M. Personal Recovery and Mental Illness: A Guide for Mental Health Professionals. Cambridge: Cambridge University Press; 2009.

[21] New Freedom Commission on Mental Health. Achieving the Promise: Transforming Mental Health Care in America. Rockville: US Department of Health and Human Services; 2003.

[22] Rose D, Lucas J. The user and survivor movement in Europe. In: Knapp M, McDaid D, Mossialos E, Thornicroft G, editors. Mental Health Policy and Practice across Europe: The Future Direction of Mental Health Care. Milton Keynes: Open University Press; 2006.

CHAPTER 9
Human and financial resources

Human resources

Human resources are the most critical asset in mental health service provision. The gradual transformation to community-based care has resulted in changes in the ways human resources have been utilized [1]. The essential changes have been a reallocation of staff from hospital to community-based service settings, the need for a new set of competencies which include recovery and rehabilitation [2], and the training of a wider range of workers, including informal community care workers, within the context of the practical needs of a country [3]. Further, in many low- and middle-income countries (LAMICs), trained psychiatrists work under conditions of heavy and relentless clinical activities, and may not have dedicated time during the week for any service development duties.

This reallocation of staff and redefining of roles, if not handled appropriately, may impact on staff well-being and increase staff burnout. Studies conducted shortly after the introduction of community mental health teams in the UK, for instance, found high levels of emotional exhaustion [4]. A further study found that about a third of assertive community treatment (ACT) staff (see Appendix A for details on ACT) reported high levels of emotional exhaustion [5]. These teams were less well resourced in terms of staff caseload size, the availability of a psychiatrist and dedicated beds, and the extent to which they worked outside office hours, and had less fidelity to the ACT model. The authors suggest that from the point of view of staff well-being, and therefore of team sustainability, "a combination of high caseload severity and limited resources and model fidelity may be inadvisable". Changes in staff allocation therefore need to be carefully planned and implemented.

Moreover, due to changing roles, confusions may arise between team members as to the roles and responsibilities of different professionals [6,7]. Staff may be confident about their own role, but may perceive that others do not understand it [8]. Core structures that have been identified as beneficial for good interprofessional working include [8]: having operational

Community Mental Health: putting policy into practice globally, First Edition. Graham Thornicroft, Maya Semrau, Atalay Alem, Robert E. Drake, Hiroto Ito, Jair Mari, Peter McGeorge, and R. Thara. © 2011 John Wiley & Sons, Ltd. Published 2011 by John Wiley & Sons, Ltd.

Table 9.1 Mental health staffing levels by income level of country (per 100 000 population). Source: WHO 2005 [1].

	Psychiatrists	Nurses	Psychologists	Social workers
Low-income settings	0.05	0.16	0.04	0.04
Lower middle-income settings	1.05	1.05	0.60	0.28
Higher middle-income settings	2.70	5.38	1.80	1.50
High-income settings	10.5	33.0	14.0	15.7

policies and meetings, sharing the same office space, clarity around roles and responsibilities, common policies, and team-building activities. Further, perceptions of interprofessional working by staff may be influenced by joint policies on documentation, risk, and supervision, though not by the presence of meetings and operational policy [8].

Data from the WHO Mental Health Atlas [33] show a tremendous human resource gap in developing countries. Low-income countries have only 0.05 psychiatrists and 0.16 psychiatric nurses per 100 000 people, which is about 200 times less than in high-income countries [1] (see Table 9.1 and Figure 9.2). Moreover, in sub-Saharan Africa, many countries have one psychiatrist, if that, for every million people, compared to 137 per million in the USA [9–12] (see Figure 9.1). Uganda, for example, had a population of 24.2 million in 2002 and 12 psychiatrists [13]. Chad, Eritrea, and Liberia have only one psychiatrist in each country, and Malawi in recent years has had none.

Furthermore, the existing training programs and facilities for mental health professionals in developing countries are largely inadequate to compensate for the shortage of professionals [14]. What is clear is that not only are the absolute levels of investment in mental health care particularly meager in low-income countries, they also invest a relatively low proportion of their total health budget (see Figure 9.3).

Another perspective on human resource development has been the increasing emphasis on integration of mental health into a primary care setting, thereby increasing access to the vast majority of the underserved. This has necessitated the training of general health staff in basic skills in mental health care, such as the detection of mental disorders, provision of basic care, and referral of complex problems to specialist care. In most developing countries, there is a need for a well-rounded generalist who is capable of coping with most psychiatric problems with little access to any mental health practitioner.

However, in many countries, continued training in primary care is still not regulated [15], or is altogether absent. Furthermore, whilst in some countries (such as many of the EU-15 countries), there have been detailed guidelines published with recommendations for the treatment of key

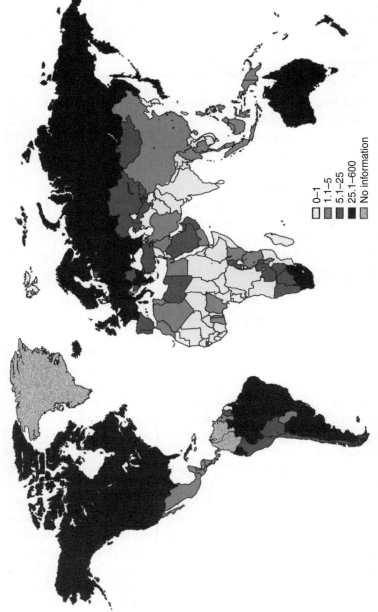

Figure 9.1 Human resources for mental health (psychiatrists, psychologists, nurses, and social workers). Source: Reprinted from Saxena et al. 2007 [14]. Copyright 2007, with permission from Elsevier.

0–1
1.1–5
5.1–25
25.1–600
No information

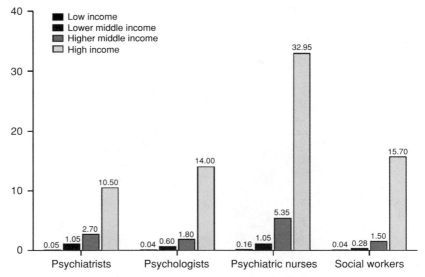

Figure 9.2 Human resources for mental health in each income group of countries per 100 000 population. Source: Reprinted from Saxena et al. 2007 [14]. Copyright 2007, with permission from Elsevier.

mental disorders in both general and specialist health settings, enabling evidence-based care—for example in the UK by the National Institute for Health and Clinical Excellence (NICE) [16]—this is often not the case in other, less resourceful countries. Further important issues are lack of insurance, out-of-pocket expenses, and the economic burden falling on families.

The broadening scope and the shift to community-based mental health services introduce greater levels of complexity, affecting the role of psychiatrists, broadening it to areas such as promotion and social inclusion. Psychiatrists therefore need to work in more settings, with more staff groups. For instance, in the Pacific Nations Islands, although fully trained mental health clinicians are employed in some nations, they are either not employed in sufficient numbers to address needs, or they are reliant on visiting specialists who do not, with few exceptions, provide adequate continuity of care for people with severe mental illnesses. Such nations rely instead on general health professionals, NGOs, and other workers such as "traditional healers" who are engaged to assist in the care of people with mental illnesses and addictions. Planning and management will take a more central place in such settings.

Psychiatrists are seen to possess a unique expertise, and occupy leading positions in most countries, functioning as advisers to governments and chairing drafting groups that are responsible for the production of policies and action plans. There are countries where such groups comprise only

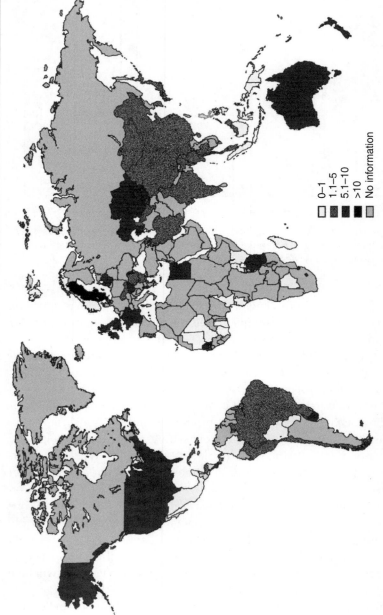

Figure 9.3 Proportion (in %) of specified budget allocated to mental health out of total health budget by country. Source: Reprinted from Saxena et al. 2007 [14]. Copyright 2007, with permission from Elsevier.

0–1
1.1–5
5.1–10
>10
No information

psychiatrists. They therefore have a unique opportunity to shape the process of reform in the best interest of patients, families, carers, the public and staff.

While psychosocial rehabilitation is an important part of the overall process of the successful management of chronic mental disorders, its practice is still rare compared to the use of medicines [17]. In many developing countries, training is scarce for occupational therapists, psychologists, and social workers. In countries with few psychiatrists, numerous medical, administrative, and leadership duties leave psychiatrists little time to work with rehabilitation units. Even so, in many LAMICs other resources are available—such as strong family and community networks, faith groups, informal employment opportunities—that might be mobilized to support the rehabilitation of people with longer-term mental disorders.

An important emerging issue in low-income settings is the concept of "task shifting". In sub-Saharan African countries, for example, where there are virtually no psychiatrists available, it is imperative that other types of staff carry out the tasks and duties traditionally reserved for psychiatrists. Further, to get the best value for the limited resources available, it will very often be necessary to allow staff with the minimum reasonable level of training to accept assessment and treatment responsibilities. This movement of tasks to less trained and less expensive staff is what is referred to as "task shifting". This approach has been applied to a series of conditions, especially infectious and communicable conditions in low-income settings [18–22], as well as a range of noncommunicable diseases [23–29], while its application to mental health care is still at an early stage [30].

Financial resources

A fundamental component in the successful implementation of mental health service provision is that of funding [31]. However, funding for mental health services in LAMICs tends to be very low [32] (see Figure 9.3). For instance, at the time of the Mental Health Atlas in eight countries (23.5%) of the Latin America and Caribbean region the total expenditure on mental health care was less than 1.0% of the total health budget. Even amongst middle- and high-income countries, such as Argentina, Brazil, and Mexico, the total expenditure was no more than 2.5% [33]. This lack of funding may be due in part to a stigmatizing attitude towards mental disorders, and to an absence of the recognition of the economic benefits that can accrue from improved mental health care. Ideally, the share of its health funding that a country devotes to mental health care will be informed by careful consideration of the comparative health benefits of spending on alternative forms of care. The data needed to carry out such an analysis are, however, typically not available in LAMICs. Furthermore, whatever funding there is also tends to be concentrated on inpatient services. One challenge is often therefore how to shift resources from these institutions to community mental health facilities. Correcting this is, initially, a matter of budgetary reallocation: using resources that could have been used for other purposes to increase funding for community-oriented care.

The issue then arises of how to pay public providers (hospitals, stand-alone programs, and possibly independent individual providers such as psychiatrists) for the services that they render. The simplest forms of payment are global budgets for facilities and programs, which may be carried over from year to year with minor adjustments for inflation, and salaries for individual providers. These simple payment mechanisms have the advantage of administrative simplicity. At the same time, they have at least two important drawbacks. First, they provide no incentive for increasing either the quantity or the quality of service provision. Second, population shifts are likely to cause the demand for the services of different providers to evolve and, without taking changes in local demand into account, inequities in payment across providers are likely to emerge and grow over time. This in turn will compromise access to overburdened providers, whilst possibly resulting in overprovision (e.g. excessive lengths of stay) by other providers. Accordingly, countries with the technical and administrative capacity to introduce more complex payment systems should consider doing so.

For hospitals, a fairly simple alternative which is applicable where care is sectorized is to modulate budgets on the basis of the population of the facility's catchment area. Countries with the technical capacity to do so may wish to adjust the payment level per person on the basis of sociodemographic variables known to be related to the need for inpatient mental health care (for example, poverty).

For hospitals that have overlapping catchment areas, a combination of prospective payment (payment on the basis of number of admissions) and retrospective payment (payment on the basis of bed days actually provided) may be preferable to exclusive reliance on one or the other. Pure retrospective payment encourages overprovision of services; pure prospective payment, given the difficulty of assessing reliably the degree of need for care of a person admitted for a psychiatric condition, may encourage underprovision.

For standalone programs or individual providers, the two main options beyond a fixed budget or a salary are fee-for-service and capitation. Fee-for-service payment encourages a higher volume of services without regard to outcomes. If certain services (e.g. prescription of medications) are paid at a higher rate per unit time than others (e.g. psychotherapy), then fee-for-service payment will also influence the mix of services provided. In addition, fee-for-service payment tends to maximize contacts with patients who are less ill, more compliant, and easier to treat. Difficult or more severely ill patients receive less care unless payments are adjusted by severity—so-called case-mix adjustments. Efficient uses of clinical time such as telephone or computer contacts are ignored because they are not reimbursed.

Capitation payment encourages increasing the number of people served. It may lead to greater accountability for the care of specific patients. In and of itself, however, unless there is competition for patients across providers, it provides no incentive for quality. Furthermore, programs often fill up to capacity and have difficulty shifting patients to less intensive services.

Countries with the technical and administrative capacity (and political leeway) to do so should consider introducing incentives for increasing quality, either for hospitals, programs, or individual providers. Following Donabedian's seminal work, quality is commonly conceptualized as related to structure, process, and outcomes [34]. Adjusting payments to hospitals, programs, or individual providers on the basis of structure or process indicators (e.g. formal qualifications of staff, achievement of a certain score on a model fidelity scale) assumes that these indicators actually predict quality. To the extent that they do, providing incentives for achieving a high score on those indicators is likely to be beneficial, with a neutral effect on which types of patient the provider will seek to serve.

Adjusting payments based on outcomes (for example, physiological indicators of metabolic syndrome, rehospitalization rates, employment rates) has the advantage of being directly related to a system's ostensible goals. It encourages, however, selection of less ill patients. More research is needed on how to design effective systems for encouraging quality of community-oriented mental health care that are practicable in countries with more- or less-developed technical and administrative capabilities.

In sum, payment systems influence patient selection, quality and amount of treatments, and outcomes, in more or less favorable ways, and different ones require varying degrees of technical and administrative capacity to be implemented successfully. Determining the optimal system or combination of systems for a particular health care setting depends heavily on history, infrastructure, financial resources, human resources, and other factors.

Key points in this chapter

- The gradual transformation to community-based care results in changes to the way that human resources are used, including a reallocation of staff from hospital to community-based service settings, the need for a new set of competencies, and training of a wider range of workers.

- Changes in staff allocation need to be carefully planned and implemented to facilitate staff well-being and avoid staff burnout.
- Having operational policies and meetings, sharing the same office space, clarity around roles and responsibilities, common policies, and team-building activities may reduce confusions by staff due to their changing roles.
- Psychiatrists' roles may broaden to areas such as promotion and social inclusion, and may include interaction with a variety of staff groups in different settings.
- In many low-resource settings there may be a need for a well-rounded generalist who is capable of coping with most psychiatric problems with little access to any mental health practitioner.
- Other resources available, such as strong family and community networks, faith groups, and informal employment opportunities, may be mobilized to support the rehabilitation of people with longer-term mental disorders.
- Task shifting, developed for infectious and communicable diseases, is beginning to be applied in mental health care.
- Funding for mental health care tends to be very limited in LAMICs (both absolutely and relatively).
- As the funding that is available in these settings is often concentrated on inpatient services, one common challenge is how to shift resources from institutions to community mental health facilities. To do so, resources that could have been used for other purposes should be utilized to increase funding for community-oriented care.
- Various payment systems are available; the most appropriate payment system for a setting may be determined by assessing its history, infrastructure, financial resources, human resources, and other factors.

References

[1] World Health Organization. Human Resources and Training in Mental Health. 2005.
[2] Slade M. Personal Recovery and Mental Illness: A Guide for Mental Health Professionals. Cambridge: Cambridge University Press; 2009.
[3] Deva PM. Training of Psychiatrists for Developing Countries. Australian and New Zealand Journal of Psychiatry 1981;15(4):343–7.
[4] Prosser D, Johnson S, Kuipers E, Dunn G, Szmukler G, Reid Y, et al. Mental health, "burnout" and job satisfaction in a longitudinal study of mental health staff. Soc Psychiatry Psychiatr Epidemiol 1999;34(6):295–300.
[5] Billings J, Johnson S, Bebbington P, Greaves A, Priebe S, Muijen M, et al. Assertive outreach teams in London: Staff experiences and perceptions. Pan-London Assertive Outreach Study, Part 2. Br J Psychiatry 2003;183:139–47.

[6] Mistral W, Hall A, McKee P. Using therapeutic community principles to improve the functioning of a high care psychiatric ward in the UK. International Journal of Mental Health Nursing 2002;11(1):10–7.

[7] Hull SA, Jones C, Tissier JM, Eldridge S, Maclaren D. Relationship style between GPs and community mental health teams affects referral rates. Br J Gen Pract 2002; 52(475):101–7.

[8] Larkin C, Callaghan P. Professionals' perceptions of interprofessional working in community mental health teams. Journal of Interprofessional Care 2005; 19(4):338–46.

[9] Miller G. Mental health in developing countries: A spoonful of medicine—and a steady diet of normality. Science 2006;311(5760):464–5.

[10] Miller G. Mental health in developing countries—China: Healing the metaphorical heart. Science 2006;311(5760):462–3.

[11] Miller G. Mental health in developing countries—Mapping mental illness: An uncertain topography. Science 2006;311(5760):460–1.

[12] Miller G. Mental health in developing countries—The unseen: Mental illness's global toll. Science 2006;311(5760):458–61.

[13] Ndyanabangi S, Basangwa D, Lutakome J, Mubiru C. Uganda mental health country profile. Int Rev Psychiatry 2004;16(1–2):54–62.

[14] Saxena S, Thornicroft G, Knapp M, Whiteford H. Resources for mental health: Scarcity, inequity, and inefficiency. Lancet 2007;370(9590):878–89.

[15] World Health Organization. Policies and Practices for Mental Health in Europe: Meeting the Challenges. 2008.

[16] National Institute for Health and Clinical Excellence (NICE). http://www.nice.org.uk/.

[17] Deva P. Psychiatric rehabilitation and its present role in developing countries. World Psychiatry 2006;5:164–5.

[18] Philips M, Zachariah R, Venis S. Task shifting for antiretroviral treatment delivery in sub-Saharan Africa: Not a panacea. Lancet 2008;371(9613):682–4.

[19] Shumbusho F, van Griensven J, Lowrance D, Turate I, Weaver MA, Price J, et al. Task shifting for scale-up of HIV care: Evaluation of nurse-centered antiretroviral treatment at rural health centers in Rwanda. PLoS Med 2009;6(10):e1000163.

[20] Babigumira JB, Castelnuovo B, Lamorde M, Kambugu A, Stergachis A, Easterbrook P, et al. Potential impact of task-shifting on costs of antiretroviral therapy and physician supply in Uganda. BMC Health Serv Res 2009;9: 192.

[21] Price J, Binagwaho A. From medical rationing to rationalizing the use of human resources for AIDS care and treatment in Africa: A case for task shifting. Dev World Bioeth 2010;10(2):99–103.

[22] Callaghan M, Ford N, Schneider H. A systematic review of task-shifting for HIV treatment and care in Africa. Hum Resour Health 2010;8:8.

[23] McPake B, Mensah K. Task shifting in health care in resource-poor countries. Lancet 2008;372(9642):870–1.

[24] De Brouwere V, Dieng T, Diadhiou M, Witter S, Denerville E. Task shifting for emergency obstetric surgery in district hospitals in Senegal. Reprod Health Matters 2009;17(33):32–44.

[25] McLaughlin PM, Borrie MJ, Murtha SJ. Shifting efficacy, distribution of attention and controlled processing in two subtypes of mild cognitive impairment: Response time performance and intraindividual variability on a visual search task. Neurocase 2010;16(5):408–17.

[26] Labhardt ND, Balo JR, Ndam M, Grimm JJ, Manga E. Task shifting to non-physician clinicians for integrated management of hypertension and diabetes in

rural Cameroon: A programme assessment at two years. BMC Health Serv Res 2010;10:339.

[27] Fulton BD, Scheffler RM, Sparkes SP, Auh EY, Vujicic M, Soucat A. Health workforce skill mix and task shifting in low income countries: A review of recent evidence. Hum Resour Health 2011;9(1):1.

[28] Hoke TH, Wheeler SB, Lynd K, Green MS, Razafindravony BH, Rasamihajamanana E, et al. Community-based provision of injectable contraceptives in Madagascar: "Task shifting" to expand access to injectable contraceptives. Health Policy Plan 2011; epub ahead of print.

[29] Gessessew A, Barnabas GA, Prata N, Weidert K. Task shifting and sharing in Tigray, Ethiopia, to achieve comprehensive emergency obstetric care. Int J Gynaecol Obstet 2011;113(1):28–31

[30] Petersen I, Lund C, Bhana A, Flisher AJ. A task shifting approach to primary mental health care for adults in South Africa: Human resource requirements and costs for rural settings. Health Policy Plan 2011; epub ahead of print.

[31] Thornicroft G, Tansella M. Components of a modern mental health service: A pragmatic balance of community and hospital care—Overview of systematic evidence. British Journal of Psychiatry 2004;185:283–90.

[32] Saraceno B, Van OM, Batniji R, Cohen A, Gureje O, Mahoney J, et al. Barriers to improvement of mental health services in low-income and middle-income countries. Lancet 2007;370(9593):1164–74.

[33] World Health Organization. Mental Health Atlas, revised edition. 2005.

[34] Best M, Neuhauser D. Avedis Donabedian: Father of quality assurance and poet. Quality and Safety in Health Care 2004;13:472–3.

CHAPTER 10

Development, organization, and evaluation of services

Developing services

The initiation of community mental health care services generally requires strong leadership among stakeholders based on community-oriented care concepts. It is practical to learn from successful models by using basic tools including timetables, assessment forms, job descriptions, and operational policies, acquired during site visits for example [1]. Coaching and maintenance activities are needed to make services robust and sustainable. It can be useful for staff in specific clinical teams to develop a manual (or standard operating procedure) for routine tasks for which operational standards have been agreed, so that ongoing supervision can assess whether these standards are met and maintained. These may be important "soft" components of consolidating a new pattern of care.

Organizational issues

Quality assurance is feasible even in settings with limited resources. Quality monitoring can be incorporated into routine activities by selecting target services, collecting data, and using the results for system problem solving and future direction. External evaluation takes place at different levels; local government checks whether service providers meet the requirement of laws or acts, while payers focus on examining the necessity of services provided. Professional peers and consumers also participate in independent evaluation.

Service evaluation

Since the primary purpose of mental health services is to improve outcomes for individuals with mental illness, it is crucial to assess outcomes

Community Mental Health: putting policy into practice globally, First Edition. Graham Thornicroft, Maya Semrau, Atalay Alem, Robert E. Drake, Hiroto Ito, Jair Mari, Peter McGeorge, and R. Thara. © 2011 John Wiley & Sons, Ltd. Published 2011 by John Wiley & Sons, Ltd.

of treatments and services [2]. The results can be used to justify the use of resources. Europe is one of the regions where there has been the most high-quality research (i.e. systematic reviews or randomized controlled trials (RCTs)) conducted on the evaluation of community mental health services, though most publications in the region stem from the UK (around 80% of studies) and a few other well-resourced countries (at least those published in English).

Research evidence from systematic reviews and RCTs evaluating community mental health services in the European region are displayed in Tables 10.1 and 10.2. Overall, this evidence suggests that, in principle, community-based mental health care is effective. There is some evidence for the effectiveness of an integration of mental health into primary health services across different models of care, as well as for community mental health teams, assertive community treatment, intensive case management, crisis intervention, and supported employment. However, high-quality evaluative evidence for other mainstream or specialized community mental health services is inconsistent or missing.

Assessment of services' comparative effectiveness is often problematic due to a lack of clarity about the model of care; that is, services described by one team often contain components of care employed by other models [3, 4]. Furthermore, the components of home treatment may overlap with standard treatment, and therefore differences in outcomes may be reduced, especially where the intensity of standard treatment may be improving over time [5]. One review addressed these problems by not differentiating between home-treatment services, but instead relating components of care to effectiveness [5]. This review, which included 18 European, 35 North American, and 2 Australian studies, suggests that, regardless of service type, regular home visiting and taking of responsibility for both health and social care are associated with reduced hospitalization.

A further issue is the sustainability of services. Of the studies outlined in Tables 10.1 and 10.2, 40% had been discontinued by the publication date of their study, and a further 25% had only survived up to five years post-publication. There were insufficient data to explain why this was the case.

Other than trials of effectiveness, there have also been some observational and qualitative studies conducted in Europe. These have shown that home treatment is viewed positively by service providers [6], and that specific community mental health services, such as women's crisis houses, are highly valued by service users [7]. A national survey of UK NHS trusts and health authorities found that 97% were in favor of the principle of providing home treatment [6]. Only 16% were doing so at the time of the survey, but 40% had plans to do so.

Although research conducted in the European region may therefore act as an example in highlighting the importance and usefulness of

Table 10.1 Overview of systematic reviews evaluating community mental health services in the European region.

Authors	Service evaluated	No. studies included	Main outcomes
Burns et al. 2001 [107]	Community care (range of services) compared to admission.	91	Benefits in terms of days hospitalized (regardless of service type). Inconclusive in terms of cost-effectiveness.
Wright et al. 2004 [108]	Community care (components of care related to effectiveness).	55	Regular home visiting and taking of responsibility for both health and social care associated with reduced hospitalization (regardless of service type).
Harkness & Bower 2009 [109]	Onsite mental health workers in primary health care (replacement model) compared to offsite mental health services.	42	Small and inconsistent reduction in number of consultations with primary care providers, psychotropic prescribing, prescribing costs, and rates of referral. No effects on prescribing or referrals in the wider patient population. Cost–benefits unclear.
Gilbody et al. 2006 [110]	Collaborative care compared to usual care.	34	No significant predictor of antidepressant use. Key predictors of depression symptom outcomes were systematic identification of patients, professional background of staff, and specialist supervision.
Malone et al. 2009 [111]	Community mental health teams compared to non-team standard care (delivered as community, outpatient, or hospital treatment).	3	Reduction in hospital admissions and number of deaths by suicide. Promoted greater acceptance of treatment.
Marshall et al. 1998 [112]	Case management compared to standard community care.	10	Increased number of patients remaining in contact with services. Greater proportion of patients hospitalized. No significant benefits on psychiatric or social variables. Cost-effectiveness inconclusive.
Marshall & Lockwood 1998 [113]	Assertive community treatment compared to standard community care, hospital-based rehabilitation, or case management.	20	Improved outcome and patient satisfaction. Reduced costs of hospital care for high users of inpatient care.

(Continued)

Table 10.1 Continued.

Authors	Service evaluated	No. studies included	Main outcomes
Burns et al. 2007 [114]	Intensive case management compared to standard care for people with serious mental disorders.	29	Small but statistically significant reduction in days spent in hospital overall, but large variation between studies. Largest effects when patients had high hospital use at baseline, and the more closely treatment adhered to principles of assertive community treatment. Setting of trial did not have effect.
Marshall & Lockwood 2006 [115]	Early intervention for psychosis.	7	Evidence of poor quality overall and studies not comparable due to different intervention approaches taken
Irving et al. 2006 [116]	Crisis intervention and resolution teams (delivered as part of an ongoing home-treatment package).	5	Reduction in admissions. May be less expensive than standard care, but more data is needed to confirm this.
Macpherson et al. 2009 [117]	Community-based residential care (24-hour staffed) compared to standard hospital care.	1	Patients more likely to use social facilities and spent more time in socially constructive facilities (such as self-care, eating with group). Study was small and of poor quality.
Marshall et al. 2003 [118]	Acute day hospital care compared to inpatient care.	9	At least one-fifth of patients admitted to inpatient care could be cared for in an acute day hospital. More rapid improvement in mental state, but not social functioning. Less expensive.

Table 10.2 Overview of randomized controlled trials (RCTs) evaluating community mental health services in the European region.

Authors	Service evaluated	Country, no. subjects	Main outcomes
Richards et al. 2008 [119]	Collaborative care compared to usual care.	UK, 114	Reduction in symptoms for depressive patients.
Killaspy et al. 2006 [120], Killaspy et al. 2009 [121], McCrone et al. 2009 [122]	Assertive community treatment compared to usual care from a community mental health team.	UK, 251	No difference in the need for inpatient care, clinical or social outcomes. More contact with patients involved, but no difference in costs. Increased client satisfaction and engagement with services.
Morrison et al. 2004 [123]	Early intervention in patients with prodromal symptoms (cognitive behavior therapy compared to monitoring only).	UK, 60	No difference in leaving the study early or transition to psychosis.
Agius et al. 2007 [124]	Assertive early intervention compared to standard community mental health team.	UK, 125	Range of benefits over three years, but study not fully randomized and patients were unusually engaged with services (so results should be treated with caution).
Petersen et al. 2005 [125], Bertelsen et al. 2008 [126]	Intensive early intervention compared to standard treatment in patients with first episode schizophrenia.	Denmark, 547	Improved clinical outcome at 2 years, but effects not sustained at 5-year follow-up. Differences in the proportion of patients living in supported housing and days in hospital supported early intervention at 5-year follow-up.

(Continued)

Table 10.2 Continued.

Authors	Service evaluated	Country, no. subjects	Main outcomes
Johnson et al. 2005 [127], Cotton et al. 2007 [128]	Crisis-resolution team (24-hour short-term care) compared to standard care in patients who were experiencing a crisis severe enough to be eligible for admission.	UK, 260	Reduction in admissions. Patients most likely to be admitted to hospital were those who were uncooperative with initial assessment, at risk of self-neglect, had a history of compulsory admission, were assessed outside usual office hours, and/or were assessed in hospital casualty departments. Increased patient satisfaction.
Priebe et al. 2006 [129]	Acute day hospital care compared to conventional wards.	UK, 260	Greater improvement in psychopathology at discharge, but not at follow-up. Higher patient treatment satisfaction at discharge and after 3 months, but not after 12 months. More expensive.
Burns et al. 2007 [130], Burns et al. 2009 [131], Catty et al. 2008 [132]	Vocational rehabilitation services (supported employment) compared to other high-quality vocational services.	UK, Germany, Italy, Switzerland, Netherlands, Bulgaria, 312	Competitive employment obtained more often, jobs kept longer and more hours worked. More unwell people helped into work. Working associated with better clinical and social outcomes at 18 months. Patients with previous work history, fewer met social needs, and better relationships with their vocational workers were more likely to obtain employment and work for longer.

Note: Where there has been a systematic review published of a particular service, only those RCTs which were conducted after the review are displayed.

high-quality evaluative studies, it also emphasizes that research conducted in low- and middle-income countries (LAMICs) worldwide is scarce (as described in Chapter 6). Most research in the region is conducted in the UK and a few other well-resourced countries. More research is therefore needed worldwide to identify and provide the best possible services that would directly link to better outcomes for those in need of care.

The Balanced Care Model

The research evidence suggests that any model relevant to the vastly differing resource levels in low-, middle-, and high-resource settings needs to be realistic to the actual resources on the ground. One schema to guide investment decisions is the Balanced Care Model (BCM) [1] (also see Chapter 1).

The BCM indicates that for *low-income settings* most of the available provision is by staff in primary health care and community settings [8–12]. This can consist of: case finding and assessment; brief talking and psychosocial treatments; and pharmacological treatments [13–15]. The very limited numbers of specialist mental health care staff (usually in the capital city and sometimes also in regional centers) are only able to provide: (i) training and supervision of primary care staff; (ii) consultation liaison for complex cases; and (iii) outpatient and inpatient assessment and treatment for cases which cannot be managed in primary care [16–20].

In *medium-income settings*, it is important to appreciate that there is still a requirement for a strong primary care level of provision, so as to address the high levels of prevalence of common mental disorders in the general population (in many countries estimated at 20–30% annual period prevalence rate) [21]. The literature from such middle-income settings, for example many of the countries of Eastern Europe and South America [22–24], indicates the modest resources usually allocated for mental health care compared with communicable diseases [25–31]. Five categories of service can be developed (see Appendix A for a description of these services):
1 Outpatient/ambulatory clinics [32–35]
2 Community mental health teams (CMHTs) [36–44]
3 Acute inpatient care [45–51]
4 Long-term community-based residential care [52, 53]
5 Work and occupation [54–60].

In *high-income settings*, superimposed upon a basic primary care system [61], and also in addition to a general adult mental health care layer of services, an additional series of specialized services can be provided, as resources allow. However, it is often the case that specialized services are developed in the absence of the first two layers of general services. This can be because advocates for a new team or service take a "component view" of treatment, rather than a "system view" of the wider pattern of care, and how the constituent parts contribute to the whole [1].

Such specialized services can be developed in the same five categories described above for medium-income settings (see Appendix A):

1 Specialized outpatient/ambulatory clinics [32]
2 Specialized CMHTs, including assertive community treatment (ACT) teams [62–67] and early-intervention teams [68–77]
3 Alternatives to acute inpatient care, including acute day hospitals [56, 78], crisis houses [79–83], and home-treatment/crisis-resolution teams [84–87].
4 Alternative types of long-stay community residential care [55,88–95].
5 Specialized forms of work and occupation [56,96–106].

Key points in this chapter

- Strong leadership is required among stakeholders to initiate community mental health services.
- Coaching, maintenance activities, manualization of procedures and materials, and ongoing supervision are needed to make services robust and sustainable.
- Quality assurance is feasible even in low-resource settings. Quality monitoring can be incorporated into routine activities. External evaluation may take place at different levels, including local governments, payers, professional peers, and consumers.
- It is crucial to assess outcomes of treatments and services, including through high-quality research, in particular systematic reviews and RCTs. Such research is still scarce in most LAMICs.
- The research literature supports the Balanced Care Model (BCM), which indicates the provision in low-income settings of (a) primary care with limited specialist services.
- In medium-resources settings, provide (a) plus (b) general adult mental health care consisting of: 1 outpatient/ambulatory clinics; 2 community mental health teams; 3 acute inpatient care; 4 long-term community-based residential care; and 5 work and occupation.
- In high-resource settings, include the provision of (a), (b), and (c) specialized services in the five service categories.

References

[1] Thornicroft G, Tansella M. Better Mental Health Care. Cambridge: Cambridge University Press; 2009.
[2] Thornicroft G, Tansella M. The Mental Health Matrix: A Manual to Improve Services. Cambridge: Cambridge University Press; 1999.

[3] Burns T, Fioritti A, Holloway F, Malm U, Rossler W. Case management and assertive community treatment in Europe. Psychiatr Serv 2001;52(5):631–6.

[4] Molodynski A, Burns T. The organization of psychiatric services. Medicine 2008; 36(8):388–90.

[5] Wright C, Catty J, Watt H, Burns T. A systematic review of home treatment services—classification and sustainability [15 refs]. Social Psychiatry & Psychiatric Epidemiology 2004;39(10):789–96.

[6] Owen AJ, Sashidharan SP, Edwards LJ. Availability and acceptability of home treatment for acute psychiatric disorders: A national survey of mental health trusts and health authority purchasers. Psychiatric Bulletin 2000 May;Vol. 24(5): 169–71.

[7] Johnson S, Bingham C, Billings J, Pilling S, Morant N, Bebbington P, et al. Women's experiences of admission to a crisis house and to acute hospital wards: A qualitative study. Journal of Mental Health 2004;13(3):247–62.

[8] Deva MP. Bringing changes to Asian mental health. International Review of Psychiatry 2008;20(5):484–7.

[9] Seloilwe ES, Thupayagale-Tshweneagae G. Community mental health care in Botswana: approaches and opportunities [20 refs]. International Nursing Review 2007;54(2):173–8.

[10] Ormel J, Von Korff M, Ustun B, Pini S, Korten A. Common mental disorders and disability across cultures: Results from the WHO Collaborative Study on Psychological Problems in General Health Care. JAMA 1994;272: 1741–8.

[11] Desjarlais R, Eisenberg L, Good B, Kleinman A. World Mental Health: Problems and Priorities in Low Income Countries. Oxford: Oxford University Press; 1995.

[12] World Health Organization. World Health Report 2001. Mental Health: New Understanding, New Hope. Geneva: WHO; 2001.

[13] Eaton J. Ensuring access to psychotropic medication in sub-Saharan Africa. African Journal of Psychiatry 2008;11(3):179–81.

[14] Van Rensburg ABRJ. A changed climate for mental health care delivery in South Africa. African Journal of Psychiatry 2009;12(2):157–65.

[15] Beaglehole R, Bonita R. Global public health: A scorecard. Lancet 2008; 372(9654):1988–96.

[16] Mubbashar M. Mental health services in rural Pakistan. In: Tansella M, Thornicroft G, editors. Common Mental Disorders in Primary Care. London: Routledge; 1999. pp. 67–80.

[17] Saxena S, Maulik P. Mental health services in low and middle income countries: An overview. Curr Opin Psychiatry 2003;16: 437–42.

[18] Njenga F. Challenges of balanced care in Africa. World Psychiatry 2002;1: 96–8.

[19] Alem A. Community-based vs. hospital-based mental health care: The case of Africa. World Psychiatry 2002;1: 99–100.

[20] Thornicroft G, Tansella M. Components of a modern mental health service: A pragmatic balance of community and hospital care—Overview of systematic evidence. Br J Psychiatry 2004;185: 283–90.

[21] Kessler RC, Chiu WT, Demler O, Merikangas KR, Walters EE. Prevalence, severity, and comorbidity of 12-month DSM-IV disorders in the National Comorbidity Survey Replication. Arch Gen Psychiatry 2005;62(6):617–27.

[22] Knapp M, McDaid D, Mossialos E, Thornicroft G. Mental Health Policy and Practice across Europe. Maidenhead: Open University Press; 2007.

[23] Semrau M, Barley E, Law A, Thornicroft G. Lessons learned in developing community mental health care. 3. Europe. World Psychiatry 2011; in press.

[24] Razzouk D, Gregorio G, Antunes R, Mari J. Lessons learned in developing community mental health care. 5. Latin American and Caribbean countries. World Psychiatry 2011; in press.

[25] Al-Krenawi A. Mental health practice in Arab countries. Current Opinion in Psychiatry 2005;18(5):560–4.

[26] Sharifi V. Urban mental health in Iran: Challenges and future directions. Iranian Journal of Psychiatry and Behavioral Sciences 2009;3(1):9–14.

[27] Furedi J, Mohr P, Swingler D, Bitter I, Gheorghe MD, Hotujac L, et al. Psychiatry in selected countries of Central and Eastern Europe: An overview of the current situation [21 refs]. Acta Psych Scand 2006;114(4):223–31.

[28] Janse van Rensburg AB. A changed climate for mental health care delivery in South Africa [65 refs]. African Journal of Psychiatry 2009;12(2):157–65.

[29] Akiyama T, Chandra N, Chen CN, Ganesan M, Koyama A, Kua EE, et al. Asian models of excellence in psychiatric care and rehabilitation [30 refs]. International Review of Psychiatry 2008;20(5):445–51.

[30] Razali SM. Deinstitutionalization and community mental health services in Malaysia: An overview. International Medical Journal 2004;11(1):29–35.

[31] Rodrguez JJ. Mental health care systems in Latin America and the Caribbean. International Review of Psychiatry 2010;22(4):317–24.

[32] Becker T, Koesters M. Psychiatric outpatient clinics. In: Thornicroft G, Szmukler GI, Mueser KT, Drake RE, editors. Oxford Textbook of Community Mental Health. Oxford: Oxford University Press; 2011. pp. 179–91.

[33] Nathan P, Gorman J. A Guide to Treatments that Work, 2nd ed. Oxford: Oxford University Press; 2002.

[34] Roth A, Fonagy P. What Works for Whom? A Critical Review of Psychotherapy Research. New York: Guildford Press; 1996.

[35] BMJ Books. Clinical Evidence, volume 9. London: BMJ Books; 2003.

[36] Thornicroft G, Becker T, Holloway F, Johnson S, Leese M, McCrone P, et al. Community mental health teams: Evidence or belief? Br J Psychiatry 1999;175: 508–13.

[37] Department of Health. Community Mental Health Teams, Policy Implementation Guidance. London: Department of Health; 2002.

[38] Tyrer P, Morgan J, Van Horn E, Jayakody M, Evans K, Brummell R, et al. A randomised controlled study of close monitoring of vulnerable psychiatric patients. Lancet 1995;345(8952):756–9.

[39] Tyrer P, Evans K, Gandhi N, Lamont A, Harrison-Read P, Johnson T. Randomised controlled trial of two models of care for discharged psychiatric patients. BMJ 1998;316(7125):106–9.

[40] Thornicroft G, Wykes T, Holloway F, Johnson S, Szmukler G. From efficacy to effectiveness in community mental health services. PRiSM Psychosis Study. Br J Psychiatry 1998;173: 423–7.

[41] Simmonds S, Coid J, Joseph P, Marriott S, Tyrer P. Community mental health team management in severe mental illness: A systematic review. Br J Psychiatry 2001;178: 497–502.

[42] Tyrer S, Coid J, Simmonds S, Joseph P, Marriott S. Community Mental Health Teams (CMHTs) for People with Severe Mental Illnesses and Disordered Personality (Cochrane Review). Oxford: Update Software; 2003.

[43] Burns T. Generic versus specialist mental health teams. In: Thornicroft G, Szmukler G, editors. Textbook of Community Psychiatry. Oxford: Oxford University Press; 2001. pp. 231–41.

[44] Sytema S, Micciolo R, Tansella M. Continuity of care for patients with schizophrenia and related disorders: A comparative south-Verona and Groningen case-register study. Psychol Med 1997;27(6):1355–62.

[45] Holloway F, Sederer L. Inpatient treatment. In: Thornicroft G, Szmukler GI, Mueser KT, Drake RE, editors. Oxford Textbook of Community Mental Health. Oxford: Oxford University Press; 2011. pp. 223–31.

[46] Johnstone P, Zolese G. Systematic review of the effectiveness of planned short hospital stays for mental health care. BMJ 1999;318(7195):1387–90.

[47] Knapp M, Chisholm D, Astin J, Lelliott P, Audini B. The cost consequences of changing the hospital–community balance: The mental health residential care study. Psychol Med 1997;27(3):681–92.

[48] Lasalvia A, Tansella M. Acute in-patient care in modern, community-based mental health services: Where and how? Epidemiol Psichiatr Soc 2010;19(4):275–81.

[49] Totman J, Mann F, Johnson S. Is locating acute wards in the general hospital an essential element in psychiatric reform? The UK experience. Epidemiol Psichiatr Soc 2010;19(4):282–6.

[50] Sederer LI. Inpatient psychiatry: Why do we need it? Epidemiol Psichiatr Soc 2010;19(4):291–5.

[51] Lelliott P, Bleksley S. Improving the quality of acute inpatient care. Epidemiol Psichiatr Soc 2010;19(4):287–90.

[52] Shepherd G, MacPherson R. Residential care. In: Thornicroft G, Szmukler GI, Mueser KT, Drake RE, editors. Oxford Textbook of Community Mental Health. Oxford: Oxford University Press; 2011. pp. 232–44.

[53] van Wijngaarden GK, Schene A, Koeter M, Becker T, Knudsen HC, Tansella M, et al. People with schizophrenia in five European countries: Conceptual similarities and intercultural differences in family caregiving. Schizophr Bull 2003; 29(3):573–86.

[54] Shepherd G. Theory and Practice of Psychiatric Rehabilitation. Chichester: Wiley; 1990.

[55] Rosen A, Barfoot K. Day care and occupation: Structured rehabilitation and recovery programmes and work. In: Thornicroft G, Szmukler G, editors. Textbook of Community Psychiatry. Oxford: Oxford University Press; 2001. pp. 296–308.

[56] Marshall M, Crowther R, Almaraz-Serrano A, Creed F, Sledge W, Kluiter H, et al. Systematic reviews of the effectiveness of day care for people with severe mental disorders: (1) Acute day hospital versus admission; (2) Vocational rehabilitation; (3) Day hospital versus outpatient care. Health Technol. Assess. 2003;5(21):1–75.

[57] Cleary M, Freeman A, Walter G. Carer participation in mental health service delivery [32 refs]. International Journal of Mental Health Nursing 2006;15(3):189–94.

[58] Slade M. Personal Recovery and Mental Illness: A Guide for Mental Health Professionals. Cambridge: Cambridge University Press; 2009.

[59] Catty J, Burns T, Comas A. Day Centres for Severe Mental Illness (Cochrane Review). The Cochrane Library, Issue 1. Oxford: Update Software; 2003.

[60] Becker DR, Bond GR, Drake RE. Individual placement and support: The evidence-based practice of supported employment. In: Thornicroft G, Szmukler GI, Mueser KT, Drake RE, editors. Oxford Textbook of Community Mental Health. Oxford: Oxford University Press; 2011. pp. 204–17.

[61] Gask L. Overt and covert barriers to the integration of primary and specialist mental health care. Social Science and Medicine 2005;61(8):1785–94.

[62] Deci PA, Santos AB, Hiott DW, Schoenwald S, Dias JK. Dissemination of assertive community treatment programs. Psychiatr Serv 1995;46(7):676–8.

[63] Teague GB, Bond GR, Drake RE. Program fidelity in assertive community treatment: Development and use of a measure. Am J Orthopsychiatry 1998;68(2): 216–32.

[64] Scott J, Lehman A. Case management and assertive community treatment. In: Thornicroft G, Szmukler G, editors. Textbook of Community Psychiatry. Oxford: Oxford University Press; 2001. pp. 253–64.

[65] Fiander M, Burns T, McHugo GJ, Drake RE. Assertive community treatment across the Atlantic: Comparison of model fidelity in the UK and USA. Br J Psychiatry 2003;182: 248–54.

[66] Burns T, Creed F, Fahy T, Thompson S, Tyrer P, White I. Intensive versus standard case management for severe psychotic illness: A randomised trial—UK 700 Group. Lancet 1999;353(9171):2185–9.

[67] Burns T, Fioritti A, Holloway F, Malm U, Rossler W. Case management and assertive community treatment in Europe. Psychiatr Serv 2001;52(5):631–6.

[68] Power P, McGorry P. Early interventions for people with psychotic disorders. In: Thornicroft G, Szmukler GI, Mueser KT, Drake RE, editors. Oxford Textbook of Community Mental Health. Oxford: Oxford University Press; 2011. pp. 159–60.

[69] Preti A, Cella M. Randomized-controlled trials in people at ultra high risk of psychosis: A review of treatment effectiveness. Schizophr Res 2010;123(1):30–6.

[70] Addington J, Coldham EL, Jones B, Ko T, Addington D. The first episode of psychosis: The experience of relatives. Acta Psychiatr Scand 2003;108(4):285–9.

[71] Raune D, Kuipers E, Bebbington PE. Expressed emotion at first-episode psychosis: Investigating a carer appraisal model. Br J Psychiatry 2004;184: 321–6.

[72] Killackey E. Review: Early intervention services can be clinically beneficial for people with early psychosis. Evid Based Ment Health 2011; epub ahead of print.

[73] Larsen TK, Melle I, Auestad B, Haahr U, Joa I, Johannessen JO, et al. Early detection of psychosis: Positive effects on 5-year outcome. Psychol Med 2010;14: 1–9.

[74] Bosanac P, Patton GC, Castle DJ. Early intervention in psychotic disorders: Faith before facts? Psychol Med 2010;40(3):353–8.

[75] Gafoor R, Nitsch D, McCrone P, Craig TK, Garety PA, Power P, et al. Effect of early intervention on 5-year outcome in non-affective psychosis. Br J Psychiatry 2010; 196(5):372–6.

[76] Marshall M, Rathbone J. Early intervention for psychosis. Cochrane Database Syst Rev 2006; (4):CD004718.

[77] Marshall M, Lockwood A. Early Intervention for psychosis. Cochrane Database Syst Rev 2004; (2):CD004718.

[78] Wiersma D, Kluiter H, Nienhuis FJ, Ruphan M, Giel R. Costs and benefits of hospital and day treatment with community care of affective and schizphrenic disorders. Br J Psychiatry Suppl 1995;27: 52–9.

[79] Sledge WH, Tebes J, Wolff N, Helminiak TW. Day hospital/crisis respite care versus inpatient care. Part II. Service utilization and costs. Am J Psychiatry 1996; 153(8):1074–83.

[80] Sledge WH, Tebes J, Rakfeldt J, Davidson L, Lyons L, Druss B. Day hospital/crisis respite care versus inpatient care. Part I. Clinical outcomes. Am J Psychiatry 1996; 153(8):1065–73.

[81] Davies S, Presilla B, Strathdee G, Thornicroft G. Community beds: The future for mental health care? Soc Psychiatry Psychiatr Epidemiol 1994;29(6):241–3.

[82] Szmukler G, Holloway F. In-patient treatment. In: Thornicroft G, Szmukler G, editors. Textbook of Community Psychiatry. Oxford: Oxford University Press; 2001. pp. 321–37.

[83] Mosher LR. Soteria and other alternatives to acute psychiatric hospitalization: A personal and professional review [48 refs]. Journal of Nervous & Mental Disease 1999;187(3):142–9.

[84] Catty J, Burns T, Knapp M, Watt H, Wright C, Henderson J, et al. Home treatment for mental health problems: A systematic review. Psychol Med 2002;32(3):383–401.

[85] Irving CB, Adams CE, Rice K. Crisis intervention for people with severe mental illnesses. Cochrane Database Syst Rev 2009; (4):CD001087.

[86] Joy CB, Adams CE, Rice K. Crisis intervention for people with severe mental illnesses. Cochrane Database Syst Rev 2006; (4):CD001087.

[87] Johnson S, Needle J, Bindman J, Thornicroft G. Crisis Resolution and Home Treatment in Mental Health. Cambridge: Cambridge University Press; 2008.

[88] Shepherd G, Muijen M, Dean R, Cooney M. Residential care in hospital and in the community—Quality of care and quality of life. Br J Psychiatry 1996; 168(4):448–56.

[89] Shepherd G, Murray A. Residential care. In: Thornicroft G, Szmukler G, editors. Textbook of Community Psychiatry. Oxford: Oxford University Press; 2001. pp. 309–20.

[90] Trieman N, Smith HE, Kendal R, Leff J. The TAPS Project 41: Homes for life? Residential stability five years after hospital discharge—Team for the Assessment of Psychiatric Services. Community Ment Health J 1998;34(4):407–17.

[91] Chilvers R, Macdonald G, Hayes A. Supported housing for people with severe mental disorders (Cochrane Review). Oxford: Update Software; 2003.

[92] Thornicroft G, Bebbington P, Leff J. Outcomes for long-term patients one year after discharge from a psychiatric hospital. Psychiatr Serv 2005;56(11):1416–22.

[93] Nordentoft M, Knudsen HC, Schulsinger F. Housing conditions and residential needs of psychiatric patients in Copenhagen. Acta Psychiatr Scand 1992; 85(5):385–9.

[94] Hafner H. Do we still need beds for psychiatric patients? An analysis of changing patterns of mental health care. Acta Psychiatr Scand 1987;75(2):113–26.

[95] Thornicroft G. Measuring Mental Health Needs, 2nd ed. London: Royal College of Psychiatrists, Gaskell; 2001.

[96] Lehman A. Vocational rehabilitation in schizophrenia. Schizophrenia Bulletin 1995;21: 645–56.

[97] Thornicroft G, Tansella M, Becker T, Knapp M, Leese M, Schene A, et al. The Personal Impact of Schizophrenia in Europe. Schizophrenia Research 2004;69: 125–32.

[98] Marwaha S, Johnson S, Bebbington P, Stafford M, Angermeyer MC, Brugha T, et al. Rates and correlates of employment in people with schizophrenia in the UK, France and Germany. British Journal of Psychiatry 2007;191: 30–7.

[99] Thornicroft G, Rose D, Huxley P, Dale G, Wykes T. What are the research priorities of mental health service users? Journal of Mental Health 2002;11: 1–5.

[100] Becker DR, Drake RE, Farabaugh A, Bond GR. Job preferences of clients with severe psychiatric disorders participating in supported employment programs. Psychiatr Serv 1996;47(11):1223–6.

[101] Bond GR, Drake RE, Becker DR. An update on randomized controlled trials of evidence-based supported employment. Psychiatric Rehabilitation Journal 2008; 31(4):280–90.

[102] Crowther RE, Marshall M, Bond GR, Huxley P. Helping people with severe mental illness to obtain work: Systematic review. British Medical Journal 2001;322(7280):204–8.

[103] Rinaldi M, Perkins R. Comparing employment outcomes for two vocational services: Individual placement and support and non-integrated pre-vocational services in the UK. Journal of Vocational Rehabilitation 2007;27(1):21–7.

[104] Drake RE, McHugo GJ, Bebout RR, Becker DR, Harris M, Bond GR, et al. A randomized clinical trial of supported employment for inner-city patients with severe mental disorders. Arch Gen Psychiatry 1999;56(7):627–33.

[105] Priebe S, Warner R, Hubschmid T, Eckle I. Employment, attitudes toward work, and quality of life among people with schizophrenia in three countries. Schizophr Bull 1998;24(3):469–77.

[106] Lehman AF, Goldberg R, Dixon LB, McNary S, Postrado L, Hackman A, et al. Improving employment outcomes for persons with severe mental illnesses. Arch Gen Psychiatry 2002;59(2):165–72.

[107] Burns T, Knapp M, Catty J, Healey A, Henderson J, Watt H, et al. Home treatment for mental health problems: A systematic review. Health Technol Assess 2001; 5(15):1–139.

[108] Wright C, Catty J, Watt H, Burns T. A systematic review of home treatment services: Classification and sustainability. Social Psychiatry and Psychiatric Epidemiology 2004;39(10):789–96.

[109] Harkness E, Bower P. On-site mental health workers delivering psychological therapy and psychosocial interventions to patients in primary care: Effects on the professional practice of primary care providers. Cochrane Database Syst Rev 2009; (1):CD000532.

[110] Gilbody S, Bower PJ, Fletcher J, Richards DA, Sutton A. Collaborative care for depression: A systematic review and cumulative meta-analysis. Archives of Internal Medicine 2006;166: 2314–21.

[111] Malone D, Marriott S, Newton-Howes G, Simmonds S, Tyrer P. Community mental health teams for people with severe mental illnesses and disordered personality. Schizopr. Bull 2009;35(1):13–14.

[112] Marshall M, Gray A, Lockwood A, Green R. Case management for people with severe mental disorders. Cochrane Database Syst Rev 1998; (2):CD000050.

[113] Marshall M, Lockwood A. Assertive community treatment for people with severe mental disorders. Cochrane Database Syst Rev 1998; (2):CD001089.

[114] Burns T, Catty J, Dash M, Roberts C, Lockwood A, Marshall M. Use of intensive case management to reduce time in hospital in people with severe mental illness: Systematic review and meta-regression. British Medical Journal 2007;335(7615):336.

[115] Marshall M, Lockwood A. Early Intervention for Psychosis. Cochrane Database Syst Rev 2006; (4):CD004718.

[116] Irving CR, Adams CE, Rice K. Crisis intervention for people with severe mental illnesses. Cochrane Database Syst Rev 2006; (4):CD001087.

[117] Macpherson R, Edwards T, Chilvers R, David C, Elliott H. Twenty-four hour care for schizophrenia. Cochrane Database Syst Rev 2009; (2):CD004409.

[118] Marshall M, Crowther R, Almaraz-Serrano A, Sledge W, Kluiter H, Roberts C, et al. Day hospital versus admissions for acute psychiatric disorders. Cochrane Database Syst Rev 2003; (1):CD004026.

[119] Richards DA, Lovell K, Gilbody S, Gask L, Torgerson D, Barkham M, et al. Collaborative care for depression in UK primary care: A randomized controlled trial. Psychological Medicine 2008;38(2):279–87.

[120] Killaspy H, Bebbington P, Blizard R, Johnson S, Nolan F, Pilling S, et al. The REACT study: Randomised evaluation of assertive community treatment in north London. BMJ 2006;332: 815–20.

[121] Killaspy H, Johnson S, Pierce B, Bebbington P, Pilling S, Nolan F, et al. Successful engagement: A mixed methods study of the approaches of assertive community treatment and community mental health teams in the REACT trial. Social Psychiatry and Psychiatric Epidemiology 2009;44: 532–40.

[122] McCrone P, Killaspy H, Bebbington P, Johnson S, Nolan F, Pilling S, et al. The REACT study: Cost-effectiveness analysis of assertive community treatment in North London. Psychiatric Services 2009;60(7):908–13.

[123] Morrison AP, Renton JC, Williams S, Dunn H, Knight A, Kreutz M, et al. Delivering cognitive therapy to people with psychosis in a community mental health setting: An effectiveness study. Acta Psychiatrica Scandinavica 2004;110: 36–44.

[124] Agius M, Shah S, Ramkisson R, Murphy S, Zaman R. Three year outcomes of an early intervention for psychosis service as compared with treatment as usual for first psychotic episodes in a standard community mental health team final results. Psychiatria Danubina 2007;19: 130–8.

[125] Petersen L, Jeppesen P, Thorup A, Abel MB, Ohlenschlaeger J, Christensen TO, et al. A randomised multicentre trial of integrated versus standard treatment for patients with a first episode of psychotic illness. British Medical Journal 2005;331(7517):602.

[126] Bertelsen M, Jeppesen P, Petersen L, Thorup A, Ohlenschlaeger J, et al. Five-year follow-up of a randomized multicenter trial of intensive early intervention vs standard treatment for patients with a first episode of psychotic illness: The OPUS trial. Arch. Gen. Psychiatry 2008;65: 762–71.

[127] Johnson S, Nolan F, Pilling S, Sandor A, Hoult J, McKenzie N, et al. Randomised controlled trial of acute mental health care by a crisis resolution team: The north Islington crisis study. BMJ 2005;331(7517): 599–602.

[128] Cotton M, Johnson S, Bindman J, Sandor A, White I, Thornicroft G, et al. An investigation of factors associated with psychiatric hospital admission despite the presence of crisis resolution teams. BMC Psychiatry 2007;7: 52.

[129] Priebe S, Jones G, McCabe R, Briscoe J, Wright D, Sleed M, et al. Effectiveness and costs of acute day hospital treatment compared with conventional in-patient care: Randomised controlled trial. British Journal of Psychiatry 2006;188: 243–9.

[130] Burns T, Catty J, Becker T, Drake RE, Fioritti A, Knapp M, et al. The effectiveness of supported employment for people with severe mental illness: A randomised controlled trial. Lancet 2007;370: 1146–52.

[131] Burns T, Catty J, White S, Becker T, Koletsi M, Fioritti A, et al. The impact of supported employment and working on clinical and social functioning: Results of an international study of individual placement and support. Schizophrenia Bulletin 2009;35: 949–58.

[132] Catty J, Lissouba P, White S, Becker T, Drake RE, Fioritti A, et al. Predictors of employment for people with severe mental illness: Results of an international six-centre randomised controlled trial. British Journal of Psychiatry 2008;192: 224–31.

SECTION 3

Recommendations

CHAPTER 11

Lessons learned and recommendations for the future

Introduction

This concluding chapter provides an overview of the challenges, lessons learned, and recommendations for the provision of mental health care. Drawing upon the literature reviewed, and our own accumulated experience, we recount a series of commonly occurring challenges and obstacles to implementing a community-oriented system of mental health care across regions worldwide. At the same time we identify related steps and solutions which may work across regions in responding positively and effectively to these barriers [1, 2]. Challenges, lessons learned, and recommendations are then discussed in turn in more detail for each region. We recommend that people interested in planning and implementing systems of mental health care which balance community-based and hospital-based service components give careful consideration to anticipating the challenges identified here, and to learning the lessons from those who have grappled with these issues so far.

Mistakes identified across regions

Several key mistakes are commonly made in the process of attempting to implement community mental health care. First, there needs to be a carefully considered sequence of events linking hospital bed closure to community service development. It is important to avoid closing hospital-based services without having successor services already in place to support discharged patients and new referrals, and also to avoid trying to build up community services while leaving hospital care (and budgets)

Community Mental Health: putting policy into practice globally, First Edition. Graham Thornicroft, Maya Semrau, Atalay Alem, Robert E. Drake, Hiroto Ito, Jair Mari, Peter McGeorge, and R. Thara. © 2011 John Wiley & Sons, Ltd. Published 2011 by John Wiley & Sons, Ltd.

intact. In particular, there needs to be at each stage of a reform process a workable balance between enough (mainly acute) beds and the provision of other parts of the wider system of care that can support people in crisis.

A second common mistake is to attempt system reform without including *all* the relevant stakeholders. Such initiatives particularly need to include psychiatrists, who may otherwise feel subject to "top-down" decision making and react, either in the interests of patients or in their own interests, by attempting to delay or block any such changes. Other vital stakeholders to be directly included in the process will often include policy makers and politicians, health service planners, service users and carers, service providers—including those in state and private practice—national and international NGOs, those working in alternative, complementary, indigenous, and religious healing traditions, and relevant national and professional associations. Typically, those groups not fully involved in a reform process will make their views known by seeking to undermine the process.

A further common mistake is to inappropriately link the reform of mental health care with narrow ideological or party-political interests. This tends to lead to instability, as a change of government may reverse the policies of the outgoing administration. Such fault lines of division or fragmentation may also occur, for example, between service reforms proposed by psychologists and psychiatrists, between socially- and biologically-oriented psychiatrists, or between clinicians and service user/consumer groups. Whatever the particular points of schism, such conflicts weaken the chance that service reforms will be comprehensive, systemic, and sustainable, and they also run the risk that policy makers will refuse to adopt proposals that are not fully endorsed by the whole mental health sector.

Additional issues that may compromise the integrity of community-based services include: (i) an exclusive focus of community services on psychotic conditions, so that the vast majority of people with mental disorders are neglected or dealt with by professionals who do not have the appropriate expertise; and (ii) the neglect of patients' physical health.

Lessons learned and recommendations across regions

Table 11.1 provides an overview of the obstacles, challenges, lessons learned, and solutions which we have identified in the implementation of community mental health care across regions worldwide.

Table 11.1 Obstacles, challenges, lessons learned, and solutions in implementing community-oriented mental health care worldwide.

	Obstacles and challenges	Lessons learned and solutions
1 Society	Disregard for, or violation of, human rights of people with mental illness.	Provide oversight by: civil society and service user groups, government inspectorates, international NGOs, professional associations.
		Increase population awareness of mental illness, the rights of people with mental illness, and available treatments.
	Stigma and discrimination, reflected in negative attitudes of health staff.	Encourage consumer and family/carer involvement in policy making, medical training, service provision (e.g. board member, consumer provider), and service evaluation (consumer satisfaction survey).
	Need to address different models of abnormal behavior.	Traditional and faith-based paradigms need to be amalgamated, blended, or aligned as much as possible with medical paradigms.
2 Government	Low priority given by government to mental health.	Government task force on mental illness should outline mission as a public health agenda.
		Mission can encompass values, goals, structure, development, education, training, and quality assurance for community-oriented mental health system from a public health perspective.
		Establish cross-party political support for the national policy and implementation plan.
		Provide effective advocacy on mental health gap, global burden of disease, impact of mental health conditions, cost-effectiveness of interventions, reduced life expectancy.
		Use WHO and other international agencies for advocacy, linking with priority health conditions and funds, positive response of untoward events.
		Identify champions within government who have administrative and financial authority.
	Absence or inappropriate mental health policy.	Advocate for and formulate policy based upon widespread consultation with the full range of stakeholder groups, incorporating a rationalized public health perspective based on population needs, integration of service components.
		Involve consumers in policy making.
	Absent, old, or inappropriate mental health legislation.	Create powerful lobby and rationale for mental health law.
		Modernize mental health law so that it is relevant to community-oriented care.
		Create a watchdog or inspectorate to oversee proper implementation of mental health law.

(Continued)

Table 11.1 Continued.

Obstacles and challenges	Lessons learned and solutions
Inadequate financial resources in relation to population level needs.	Help policy makers to be aware of the gap between the burden of mental illness and allocated resources, and that effective treatments are available and affordable.
	Advocate for improved mental health expenditure using relevant information, arguments, and targets, e.g. global burden of disease, mhGAP unmet needs.
	Recruit key political and governance champions to advocate for adequate funding of initiatives.
Lack of alignment between payment methods and expected services and outcomes.	Design a system that directly relates required service components and financially reimbursable categories of care, e.g. for evidence-based practices.
	Provide small financial incentives for valued outcomes.
	Create categories of reimbursement consistent with system strategy.
	Develop and use key performance indicators.
Need to address infrastructure.	Reserve transitional cost to reallocate hospital staff to community.
	Government should plan and finance efficient use of buildings, essential supplies, electronic information systems etc. to direct, monitor, and improve the system and outcomes.
Need to address structure of community-oriented service system.	Design the mental health system from local primary care to regional care to central specialty care and fill in gaps with new resources as funding grows.
Inadequate human resources for delivery of mental health care in relation to the level of need in the population.	Assess population-level needs for primary care and specialist mental health care services.
	Build capacity of health workers engaged in providing general health care and mental health care in community.
	Train current health and mental health professionals in community-oriented mental health care.
Brain-drain, failure to retain talent, staff retention, and weak career ladders.	UN agencies/international NGOs should assure sustainability of their projects/programs.
	Create exchange programs between countries.
	Create a set period of time in which medical students/registrars have to serve in their countries or rural area.
	Provide task shifting/function differentiating of psychiatrists to ensure use of their ability in their area of specialty.

	Create financial incentives and reputation systems for psychiatrists who engage in community mental health.
	Train other (less "brain-drainable") health professionals to deliver mental health care.
	Attach payment for education to the allocation and preservation of resources in order to address equitable distribution, and to prevent emigration without appropriate reimbursement.
Nonsustainable, parallel programs by international NGOs.	Close relations with ministries and other stakeholders and international NGOs.
	Put a mental health plan in place, so NGOs can help achieve its goals sustainably.
	Make sure government is proactive in collaborating with NGOs and private–public partnership.
3 Organization of the local mental health system	
Need to design, monitor, and adjust organization of mental health system.	This includes plan for local, regional, and central mental health services based on public health need, full integration with primary care, rational allocation of multidisciplinary workforce, development of information technology, funding, and use of existing facilities. All stakeholder groups can be involved in developing, monitoring, and adjusting plan.
	Set implementation plan with clear coordination between services.
	Develop policy/implementation plan with number of service needed per head of population.
	Differentiate the role of the hospital, community, and primary care services, and private and public services, using a catchment area/capitation system with a flexible funding system.
	Prioritize target groups, especially people with severe and persistent mental illness.
Lack of a feasible mental health program or nonimplementation of mental health program.	Make program highly practical by identifying resources available, tasks to be completed, allocation of responsibilities, time scales, reporting and accountability arrangements, and progress monitoring/evaluation systems.
	Have planners and professional leaders design 5 and 10 year plans.
Need to specify developmental phases.	Improve awareness of benefits of facilities and services.
Poor utilization of existing mental health facilities.	Specify pathways to care.
	Build in monitoring of quality of care, especially of process and outcome phases.

(Continued)

Table 11.1 Continued.

	Obstacles and challenges	Lessons learned and solutions
	Need to include non-medical services.	Include families, faith-based social services, NGOs, housing services, vocational services, peer-support services, and self-help services. All stakeholders involved in designing system.
		Move key tasks such as initial assessment and prescribing using a limited and affordable formulary to specially trained staff who are available at the appropriate local level.
		Identify leaders to champion and drive the process.
		Create more involvement in planning, policy making, and leadership and management.
	Lack of multisectoral collaboration, e.g. with traditional healers, housing, criminal justice, or education sectors.	Develop clear policy/implementation plan by all stakeholders.
		Collaborate with other local services to identify and help people with mental illness.
		Provide information/training to all practitioners.
		Establish multisectoral advisory and governance groups.
		Set up familiarization sessions between practitioners in the Western and local traditions.
	Poor availability or erratic supplies of psychotropic medication.	Educate policy makers and funders about the costs/benefits of specific medications.
		Provide infrastructure for clozapine monitoring.
		Monitor prescribing patterns of psychotropic medication.
		Create drug-revolving funds, public–private partnerships.
4 Professionals and practitioners	Need for leadership.	Psychiatrists and other professionals need to be involved as experts in planning, education, research, and overcoming inertia and resistance in the local environment.
	Difficulty sustaining in-service training/adequate supervision.	Provide training of trainers by staff from other regions or countries.
		Shift some psychiatric functions to trained and available practitioners.
		Lobby hard to ensure this is a priority and integral to the mental health plan.
		Introduce recovery-oriented services.
		Collect case examples of recovery.
	High staff turnover and burnout, or low staff morale.	Build trust by involving staff leaders in oversight and decision-making committees.
		Sponsor social events to enable staff to team build in non-work situations.
		Emphasize career-long continuing-training programs.
		Train supervisors.
		Provide opportunities for attending out-of-area professional meetings.
		Equip staff with sufficient skills and support.

	Poor quality of care/concern about staff skills.	Provide ongoing training and supervision.
		Create and disseminate guidelines for professionals.
		Cultivate psychiatrists' clinical skills, so that they are preserved in spite of the variety of new commitments.
		Provide third-party evaluation.
		Encourage and reward quality through awards and similar processes.
	Professional resistance, e.g. to community-oriented care and service-user involvement.	Collaborate with government and professional societies to promote the importance of community-oriented care and service-user involvement.
		Provide task shifting/function differentiating of psychiatrists to enable them to use their abilities more broadly in their area of specialty and to work with a range of stakeholders, including consumers and carers/families.
		Develop training in recovery-oriented psychosocial rehabilitation as part of training of new psychiatrists, including at medical schools in low- and middle-income countries (LAMICs).
		Collect case examples of recovery and successfully implemented community mental health initiatives.
	Dearth of relevant research to inform cost-effective services and lack of data on mental health service evaluation.	Provide more funding for research, to collect both qualitative and quantitative evidence of successfully implemented examples of community-oriented care.
	Failure to address disparities (e.g. by ethnic, economic groups).	Make sure all key stakeholders are involved.
5 Users, families, and other advocates	Need for advocacy.	Advocate for under-represented groups to develop policies and implementation plans.
		Users and other advocates may be involved in all aspects of social change, planning, lobbying the government, monitoring the development and functioning of the service system, and improving the service system.
	Need for self-help and peer-support services.	Users to lead these movements.
	Need for shared decision making.	Users and other advocates must demand at all levels that the system shifts to value the goals of users and families, and that shared decision making becomes the norm.
		Continuing professional education on human rights and staff attitudes, emphasizing attention to the preferences of consumers and carers.

Box 11.1   Factors favoring successful implementation of community mental health care in the Africa region.

- government commitment, existence of a mental health policy and legislation
- WHO support
- achieving collaboration between stakeholders
- mental health coordinator at the local level
- ongoing training and supervision
- ongoing monitoring and evaluation
- relentless networking and advocacy

Africa

Factors contributing to the success of community mental health care

Expert respondents in the survey we conducted (see Chapter 1 for details) were generally guarded about the success of implementing community mental health care in their respective countries. However, where progress had been made, a number of factors favoring success were identified, as outlined in Box 11.1.

Most respondents highlighted the importance of governmental commitment towards community mental health care in order to achieve successful implementation. The existence of national mental health policies and relevant legislation was also seen as vital, endorsed by respondents from Kenya, South Africa, Tanzania, and Uganda. Support from international agencies, particularly the World Health Organization (WHO), was also valued, both in terms of providing technical expertise and in assisting advocacy at the governmental level. Respondents emphasized the value of gaining good collaboration between all relevant stakeholders in the development of community mental health services, favoring a participatory approach for longer-term success. For example:

> We managed to co-ordinate all persons/institutions taking charge of all the components of mental health care. (Niger)

Coordination and oversight of efforts on the ground was considered by many to be a critical factor in success. In a WHO case study in South Africa, having a mental health coordinator at the district level was found to be necessary to ensure a reliable supply of psychotropic medication [3].

Important ingredients in the successful CBM community mental health program in Nigeria include ongoing and repeated training of all staff involved in the detection of persons with mental illness and delivery of mental health care, together with *"ongoing supervision, advice, monitoring and evaluation of work"*. In this project, the provision of seed money to support a drug-revolving fund helped to improve the reliability of psychotropic medication supplies. In Uganda, a similar emphasis on training of health workers at all levels, and provision of supervision by specialists, was felt to be a factor enabling success [4].

The need for relentless networking and advocacy in order to successfully implement programs was a recurring theme. As well as creating political will to support implementation, such activities are likely to be critical to underpinning the necessary conceptual change from hospital-based to community-based services. For example, successful implementation of the CBM community mental health project in Nigeria required:

> Networking with colleagues in the health service/civil service and encouraging a
> more public health approach that breaks the pattern of continuing as we have been
> going for the last few decades. (CBM, Nigeria)

On the basis of experience in providing community-based mental health care in seven low- and middle-income country (LAMIC) settings, including four from sub-Saharan Africa (Ghana, Kenya, Tanzania, and Uganda), the NGO BasicNeeds has published a report including seven features that they consider to be essential for successful scaling-up of community mental health practice [5]. These echo many of the recommendations made above, namely the importance of: community-focused government policy, dependable funding, establishment of a local management structure, appropriately adequate human resources, active user and caregiver participation, a network of stakeholders, and local context adaptations.

Some factors in the initial success of the Botswanan national program of integration of mental health into primary health care were said to include the strength of the preexisting primary health care infrastructure, commitment from the Ministry of Health, support from the WHO, and the provision of transport and accommodation for outreach clinics [6, 7]. The model of integration has also been commended, focusing as it does on close collaboration between mental health specialists and primary health care workers, without any expectation that primary health care workers would become "psychiatrically self-sufficient" [8].

Challenges in implementing community mental health care

The gap between services outlined in mental health policies and the actual implementation of community mental health care on the ground was highlighted by survey respondents from most countries. Commonalities in the kinds of challenge being faced across the African continent were evident. These are outlined in Box 11.2.

Box 11.2   Challenges in the implementation of community mental health care in the Africa region.

- competing priorities
- waning community engagement
- reliance on community volunteers (not sustainable)
- under-funding
- paucity of mental health professionals
- negative attitudes to mental health
- concern about skills of staff and quality of care
- difficulty sustaining in-service training
- erratic supplies of psychotropic medication
- lack of multisectoral collaboration, including traditional healers
- escalating need and demand for services

Although the case for developing community mental health care may be accepted at the start (albeit following intensive lobbying and awareness-raising), maintaining the focus and commitment of policy makers and health workers alike amidst the many competing priorities can be a daunting task. For example, in Liberia:

> There are so many competing priorities with very limited resources in a post conflict transitional state like ours. The high rate of poverty, illiteracy rate, extremely high infant and maternal mortality all initially caused mental health to be sidelined. (Liberia)

Participation at the community level may similarly wane over time:

> Community involvement has not been encouraging, perhaps because of competing demands of other emergencies. (Tanzania)

Programs built on the efforts of community-based volunteers may be particularly difficult to sustain in the longer-term, as such personnel are likely to seek other opportunities for career development and remuneration.

The challenge of erratic supplies of psychotropic medication can undermine an entire community mental health program, leading to loss of confidence from patients, compromised clinical care, and unaffordable out-of-pocket costs if patients are then forced to purchase medication through private vendors [5].

Under-funding of mental health care, and in particular the lack of ring-fenced money to develop mental health services, was seen as a major constraint to the implementation of services.

The chronic shortage of specialist mental health professionals to provide pre-service and in-service training and ongoing supervision of primary health care workers was seen as especially problematic. In Tanzania, typical of most sub-Saharan African countries, the availability of mental health workers was described as *"woefully inadequate"*. Even where primary health care workers receive training in mental health, there was a concern about their level of skill and the quality of care being provided (Nigeria). At times, stigmatizing attitudes towards mental health held by health workers and officials could block service development.

In Kenya, the demand and need for mental health care was perceived to be increasing, putting strain on already-stretched services. In other settings (such as Ethiopia), the reverse problem of under-utilization of biomedical mental health services was seen as a challenge, sometimes leading health service managers to question the need for expansion of services.

In practice, maintaining multisectoral collaborations was seen to be a challenge, with one adverse consequence being a narrower medical model of mental health care (for instance, without input from traditional healers or service users, or with lesser emphasis on social interventions such as income-generating activities), and a weakened voice for advocacy.

Concern that an integration of mental health care into general primary health care services will result in the further marginalization of persons with severe mental illness and a deterioration in the quality of care has also been expressed [9].

Lessons learned from the experience of implementation

On the whole, expert respondents in the Africa region reflected positively on their experiences of attempting to implement community mental health care (see Box 11.3). This was coupled with a sense that giving up was not an option given the huge gap between the burden of mental disorder and the availability of mental health care in the existing centralized, hospital-based systems.

Box 11.3   Lessons learned in implementing community mental health care in the Africa region.

- it can be done
- patience, perseverance, and determination are necessary
- sustainability requires making best use of existing systems
- allies should be identified and cultivated for support
- advocacy and community groups can influence policy makers
- supervision of primary health care (PHC) workers is necessary
- proper planning is important
- evaluation and monitoring must be integrated
- marginalization of mental health can block progress

The major lesson is that it can be done. A sizeable proportion of patients will not be reached as long as services remain exclusively provided by tertiary and secondary health facilities. (Nigeria)

With that in mind, several experts encouraged patience, perseverance, and determination. Whilst progress might be slow, and obstacles were inevitable, changes could be effected to the benefit of patients and their families.

In developing countries, the issue is so complicated, but we have to persevere. (Sudan)

In a similar spirit, much advice was directed towards the benefits to be gained over the longer term from strengthening lobbying power for mental health.

Build alliances with those who share your goals and work with them to present strong messages that cannot be ignored . . . develop relationships, and develop high quality services where results speak for themselves. (Nigeria)

Similarly,

Strategic community engagement overshadows policy makers. (Kenya)

Pragmatism was evident in experts' responses, with the recommendation of using local resources to the full, and integrating any new programs into the existing health system to ensure sustainability.

Pilot projects/NGO activities need to be integrated into the existing primary health care system, otherwise they will stall once the initial funding finishes. (Liberia)

The importance of comprehensive planning ahead of implementation was well-recognized by respondents:

Patiently planning in time and use of NGOs all help to reduce the challenges. (Uganda)

Furthermore, supervision of workers delivering mental health care, and monitoring and evaluation of the quality of care delivered, need to be an integral part of the program:

Implementation needs to be well planned, managed and evaluated. Supervision and evaluation should be built in. (South Africa)

Recommendations for the Africa region

The Africa region, with all its social, cultural, and political diversity, cannot be reduced to a single entity. Therefore our recommendations should be taken as a general framework from which individual countries can identify specific measures of relevance to their specific context.

The new impetus given to scaling up of mental health services across LAMICs [10, 11] has yet to manifest in terms of published evaluation studies establishing the effectiveness of such services in Africa. Nonetheless, an opportunity exists to build on the decades of experience, originally initiated by the WHO [12], and the existing evidence base in order to successfully implement models of community mental health care across Africa. Once stakeholders are engaged and political will is present, clear messages emerging from the evidence and experience to date support the importance of:

- Strengthening specialist mental health services whilst simultaneously integrating mental health into primary health care.
- Increasing the quality and sustainability of mental health in primary health care through adequate supervision, ongoing on-the-job training, and reliable referral networks.
- Developing robust mechanisms to ensure reliable supplies of psychotropic medications.
- Supporting the provision of simple and feasible psychosocial interventions to augment medication approaches in the time-pressed primary health care setting.
- Evaluative research that considers:
  - How the interface between primary and secondary health services affects delivery of mental health care.
  - Standardized and systematic assessments of the clinical and social outcomes of individual patients.
  - Innovative service models, including collaboration with traditional healers and religious leaders.
  - Comparative studies evaluating the relative cost-effectiveness of differing models of community care.

Australasia and South Pacific

Lessons learned across the region vary, from those related to the processes of deinstitutionalization and community development in Australasia, to the establishment of a basic infrastructure in the Pacific Nations.

Australasia

There is no question that whilst discontent about access to services and discontinuity of care are still evident, mental health services in Australia and New Zealand have been transformed over the past 20 years in terms of their mode of service delivery. They are now largely community-based and increasingly recovery-oriented. There is also a growing emphasis on consumer and family/carer involvement in service development and delivery, cultural specificity, a "whole of life" approach, and reliance on evidence-based initiatives.

Arguably, progress towards these outcomes has been more marked in New Zealand than in Australia. However, in both countries lessons have been learned in the process of transformational change. In general terms, these relate to the recognition that the development of community-oriented services is a long-term challenge which requires an intricate and sustained mix of tenacity, courage, creativity, positive relationships, good will, and good fortune to succeed.

Australasian literature relating to the change process itself is surprisingly limited. However, the various reports referred to throughout this book give some insight into the processes that have led to successful implementation and the challenges that are still to be overcome in developing a truly community-oriented system of mental health care.

The following issues cover the most important lessons learned thus far in Australia and New Zealand about what is required for the change process to succeed:

A sustained incremental approach over decades

When the psychiatric hospitals began to be closed in the 1980s, it was widely believed in Australasia that the process would be relatively straight-forward; it was simply a matter of defining patient needs and developing community-based alternatives to meet them, such as accommodation, work opportunities, social networks, and clinical care. Whilst progress has been substantial in some areas, experience overall has shown that the challenges involved are by no means linear in their nature or easily overcome. The complexity of processes ranges from the interpersonal to societal and bureaucratic, including a lack of commitment by governments to sustained and demonstrable change. In some cases, the latter has amounted to frank resistance by some politicians, professionals, and the public alike.

Given the concerns and criticisms raised in the media and literature, it is likely to be several decades before the original vision for community-oriented care can be achieved. For this, a long-range view is required which defines the ongoing challenges and ways of meeting them on a systematic and sustained basis.

Cross-party political support

In both Australia and New Zealand bipartisan political support has been given to the National Mental Health policies and plans; however, this has been translated into practice differently in the two countries, and also within the various states and territories in Australia. In New Zealand, the left-wing Labour government of the late 1980s "kick-started" the change process with its landmark first Mason enquiry into Psychiatric Services and its support for the first National Mental Health Plan. The right-wing National Party, with the personal support of its then Prime Minister Jenny Shipley, accelerated the process several fold when it came into power in the early 1990s.

Time has revealed that left-wing and right-wing support of a recovery-oriented, community-based system of care was occasioned by radically different philosophies, based respectively on notions of the collective and the individual. Nevertheless, the outcome on mental health services was significant in terms of advancing deinstitutionalization and the development of community services. To some extent, the latter process was also responsible for the progress made in Victoria, Australia; however, where progress has been more limited, the lack of coherent policy commitment has been evident.

Advocates of community care should be mindful of lobbying the support of those at all stations of the political spectrum. This involves being seen as apolitical and being prepared to support parties who promise to deliver the best deal for mental health. They should then publicly challenge, as have Professors McGorry and Hickie in Australia, other parties whose manifesto falls short, to match or exceed those offering the best deal.

Funding that is "ring-fenced"

In New Zealand, two critical features of the change process were the development of the Mental Health Commission's "Blueprint" (also see Chapter 3), and the implementation of a "funder–provider" split in the health system. The former provided a framework for funding decisions, while the latter provided the means, with government commitment to rebuilding the system following the second enquiry into Mental Health Services by Judge Ken Mason.

Funding in New Zealand has been "ring-fenced". That is, once allocated it cannot be used for any other purpose than that related to mental health care. While there have been reports of District Health Boards either under-funding mental health services or using mental health funding for other purposes, in general the ring fence has worked well in protecting the additional funds allocated to development.

Over recent years the Blueprint has began to lose relevance, as District Health Boards have adapted their funding frameworks to better meet local conditions and need. To some extent this was to be expected. However, as the process is unfolding, arbitrary forces within District Health Boards, such as a shifting of funding away from NGOs and from mental health to acute general health, may undermine the considerable gains made in developing community care.

In several Australian jurisdictions mental health funding is "quarantined". While it has been more difficult to monitor the allocation and protection of funding there than in New Zealand, there have been some beneficial effects in supporting the development of community mental health services.

In regards to the funder–provider split established in New Zealand, it is doubtful whether progress towards a recovery-oriented community-based system of care could have been achieved without it. Not only were funders more able to independently identify needs, but they were able to address those needs by funding innovative nonclinical models of care to an extent unrivalled by many other countries, and certainly Australia.

In an ideal situation, therefore, a funder–provider split and ring-fenced funding based on a template such as New Zealand's Blueprint is more likely to result in the successful implementation of community care than other traditional systems that have kept funders and providers together. The result has been that established providers tend to keep being funded, rather than innovative solutions being found to persistent challenges.

Planning that is accompanied by costed and scheduled implementation plans and mechanisms to hold agencies accountable for achieving results

Until the authority of the Mental Health Commission was weakened in 2007, under its previous legislation it was able to require costed and scheduled mental health plans to be submitted to it and in turn to the Ministry of Health on an annual basis. These detailed how additional monies allocated to the District Health Boards were to be spent and how they aligned with the Blueprint. Boards were then held accountable for the progress they had made against the Blueprint by a process of annual monitoring and the publishing of regular reports by the Commission.

In Australia, national mental health plans are produced at a very high level and as a result have been criticized for simply being aspirational and lacking the practical detail to specify funding decisions and to hold funding bodies and providers to account. To correct this and in the wake of the Mental Health Council of Australia and Senate Report on Mental Health, the Council of Australian Governments in 2006 met and produced an "Action Plan" that specified initiatives to be undertaken at a national and jurisdictional level, with funding allocated to particular areas of mental health service development.

More recently, plans have been launched by the federal government to bring the funding and management of health services together, which should benefit community mental health, as long as the principles enunciated in this volume are followed.

The importance of service champions as leaders of change

Given the complexity of the systems and the multiplicity of attitudes adopted by various stakeholders involved, visionary, skilful, and tenacious leadership in the change process can mean the difference between success and failure. Such leaders need to have a clear idea of what it is they want to achieve, the means by which this can occur, and to be able to communicate with others in ways that will convince them to support their initiative.

It is important to realize that leadership comes in various forms, each of which may be more or less important depending on the stage of the change process, and the particular issues needing to be addressed at the time. In the early stages, charismatic leadership is often required to kick-start the process. Such leaders may change their approach over time or may be replaced by quieter, more methodical—albeit no less determined—leaders who are able to organize the systems and people required to embed change. Leaders may operate at different levels and parts of the system representing different interests, whether they be clinic-, consumer-, or carer-related, but nevertheless contributing to service development as a whole. What is important overall is that there is a coherent drive towards a defined end, with each playing their part and organizing the energies of those they are leading.

Understanding the specificities of local communities and how to engage community support

There was considerable naivety displayed by those involved in the deinstitutionalization process in both Australia and New Zealand in that there was the expectation that people with mental illnesses would be welcomed back into their communities. In fact, with a few exceptions resistance has been considerable and attitudes extremely hostile. The situation, fanned by the media, stirred up fears and shored up resistance.

In some instances early and systematic consultation with neighbors enabled community-based accommodation for people with mental illnesses to be established. However, in others success was only possible by insisting on the rights of the mentally ill to be part of the community and proceeding with the establishment of residences against resistance. The lesson from these experiences is that fear and hostility, some of which involves the anticipation of losing equity because of fears of lowering property values, are common reactions when communities feel their status quo is being threatened.

However, incidents that occur in the community are likely to feed its more primitive fears and to be exploited by a media that has little regard for facts or context. To ensure forward movement in the development of community care requires such incidents to be expeditiously and properly risk managed. In this regard, the employment of people with expertise in the media and public relations can be invaluable to implementation teams.

Notwithstanding these concerns, there are people in all communities who are not only tolerant of those with mental illnesses, but actively sympathetic towards them. It is important to identify such people and to establish alliances with them early in the change process. Having done so, it is then important to be careful not to jeopardize relationships with them or in turn the relationships they have with others in their community, unless all the facts and consequences have been carefully considered.

Expertise in and commitment to models of collaborative care

In the drive to close the old psychiatric hospitals, the challenges of managing a devolved, pluralistic system and maintaining continuity of care were often not sufficiently acknowledged until too late in the process. The result has been that not knowing how to access care is still one of the most frequent complaints made by the public about mental health services, whilst disruptions to care with multiple providers is all too frequent. It is no accident that many suicides in Australasia have been commonly associated with transfers of care between providers.

In New Zealand integration has up until recently relied on goodwill between providers rather than established incentives contracted on the basis of joint care delivery with stated obligations. The initial argument was that the "market" would sort out the system and that integration would take place on the basis of mutual interest, whilst poorly performing providers would drop out of the field. In fact, the market was not strictly applied, and to the extent that it was, did not have specific contractual means to ensure integration providers became siloed.

The reliance on funding "pilots" and/or short-term contracts also complicated what otherwise would have been opportunities to find ways of developing collaborative networks of providers over longer periods of time. Ideally, care pathways mapping what providers within a locality offer people with particular conditions, and which indicate linkages and understandings between them, should be established and accessible to clinicians, service users, and families/carers alike.

Whilst governance mechanisms for integrated community systems are still being developed, having at least a rudimentary "heads of agreement" between key providers and stakeholders is crucial to beginning to meet the standards for continuity of care.

Broad-based coalitions leading to a mandated process of transparent consultation

In New Zealand, the value of a broad-based coalition for change was demonstrated. This was established under the umbrella of the New

Zealand Mental Health Foundation and came to include prominent consumer and family advocates, key NGO representatives, professional bodies, and prominent clinicians.

There is no doubt that a series of major incidents and enquiries created an impetus for changing the existing system in the late 1980s. However, the concomitant growth of the service-user movement, the establishment of mental health-specific NGOs, and Australian examples of community mental health care provided a conceptual and practical basis for shifting to a community-based system, and one which the coalition came to support. In Australia, various examples of coalitions have influenced the development of community-based care. These include peak bodies established by government to advise on development priorities to the Mental Health Council of Australia and the Mental Health Services conference (Inc) of Australia and New Zealand (THEMHS).

The new generation of service-user and family/carer advocates that have established themselves over the past three decades has been crucial to the change process. Not only have they pointed to the shortcomings and abuses of the large institutions, they have demanded and by various means influenced higher standards of care involving local access to services, home-based treatment, less compulsion, peer-support services, and their participation in service development and delivery.

Their stories have highlighted their experience of services in ways such that even those most resistant to community care have found it hard to deny the imperative for change. Although some groups may pose challenges in terms of their advocating for mental health systems that do not involve psychiatric treatments or even mental health clinicians, as part of a coalition for change their voices are arguably the most significant in effecting innovative change.

In New Zealand, the Mental Health Commission is mandated to undertake an ongoing process of consultation with the full range of agencies and groups involved in mental health care, from service users, families, clinicians, managers, and funders, to policy developers and regulators. In addition, District Health Boards and NGOs undertake regular consultative processes with their communities and stakeholders.

In Australia, consultative processes have accompanied the development of reports on progress with the National Mental Health Plan and the review of the National Mental Health Standards. Consultation with service users and their families has been undertaken by the Australian Governments Senate Committee for Mental Health and the Mental Health Council of Australia. However, while consultative processes are also built into various initiatives undertaken by State Health Departments and Public Mental Health Services, such processes tend to be conducted on a relatively ad hoc basis.

Although this may be difficult to achieve, to really effect change that reflects the gap between what is provided and what is required needs an ongoing, regular, and systematic process of consultation with stakeholders built in at several levels within the system.

Workforce

Community-based care needs a broader range of skills than that based on the requirements of hospital and outpatient clinics. Despite proclamations that clinical skills would not be required in a truly community-based system of mental health care, professionals with specialist clinical skills are essential. This said, clinicians working in the community need to have opportunities to learn new ways of thinking about, communicating, and delivering mental care in the community. This includes matters referring to building relationships with community providers, visiting service users in their own homes, working with families, community perspectives concerning mental illness, and supporting the ways people can actually live in the community. The workforce challenges occasioned by having to recruit a whole range of new clinicians to fill expanded community posts have been an extraordinary experience, particularly in New Zealand, where in one District Health Board a mental health manager's budget increased from 25 million to 52 million over the course of four years.

To address this need, major recruitment and training campaigns were undertaken and expanded to include not only a search for people with the requisite clinical skills, but also those with more generic skills to address the needs of NGO recruitment and service delivery.

Workforce substitution has begun with psychologists and nurses substituting for psychiatrists, and in turn nurse assistants substituting for nurses. In addition, special mental health diploma courses have been established to provide for the needs of people working in NGOs. Peer-support (service-user run) services are also growing at a substantial rate, especially in New Zealand.

Given the knowledge that has been acquired to date in Australasia, it would be important, in areas where deinstitutionalization is commencing or where community development has stalled, to embark on a process of establishing position and training professionals and nonprofessionals alike to fulfill the spectrum of skills required for a comprehensive system of mental health care.

Service evaluation and quality improvement

Experience in Australasia has shown that the beachhead gained by community mental health services has to be held by the establishment of systemic quality improvement mechanisms, consumer and carer participation, and service evaluation.

Ways of developing a process of continuous quality improvement are still evolving in Australasia. National Mental Health Standards in both countries have been developed and are being audited, albeit unevenly. It is evident however that a comprehensive approach to quality requires a suite of approaches rather than reliance on the implementation of national standards.

Quality improvement systems should include audit by both accreditation agencies of overall systems and providers of specific policies and procedures. The development of innovative approaches to quality improvement should also be supported and acknowledged by the establishment of "award" systems to recognize outstanding efforts.

Finally, the recognition of the importance of service evaluation requires much greater recognition in terms of funding and the part that it can play in the overall improvement of national and local service delivery systems.

Pacific Nations

The WHO initiative PIMHnet (see Chapters 4 and 5) provides the best and most recent overview of the status of mental health services in the Pacific Island Nations. In describing the presence of national policies, programs, services, and needs for workforce development it points to gaps that require addressing. It also indicates ways in which development should proceed in recommending a mixture of local initiatives supported by specialist consultant input from other countries such as Australia and New Zealand.

In the Pacific, the challenges involve education about the recognition of mental illnesses and changing attitudes to them in terms of clinical management. Beyond this, there are serious issues relating to the resourcing and prioritization of mental health services that affect the establishment of policy and plans for their development.

Lessons learned thus far relate to the importance of:

- Governments being encouraged to develop national policies and plans to address the needs of those with serious mental illnesses, based on models of community care.
- This occurring in tandem with educational efforts to increase the understanding of local people's knowledge of mental illness and what can be done to help their family members who have developed mental illnesses.
- Educational opportunities for general health professionals to gain and upskill their knowledge and practice in the recognition and treatment of mental illness.
- Making it possible for visiting specialist mental health professionals to provide consultation-liaison support for generally trained health professionals.

- Acknowledging and engaging the input of traditional healers and family members.
- Encouraging the development of mental health care pathways and referral systems.

Such initiatives need to be built on a collaborative basis from the bottom up and to involve local people wherever possible. Only by doing so will Pacific Nations have the opportunity to develop mental health services that are appropriate to their cultures, their needs, and their aspirations. This approach is crucial in ensuring that the vision of PIMHnet is achieved. The risk is that initiatives such as that sponsored by the WHO and implemented by PIMHnet will otherwise simply be seen as another version of colonization.

Europe

We present next an overview of the lessons learned in the implementation of community mental health services across Europe, as well as recommendations for the region in the future.

Treatment gap

Clinical experience and research evidence have shown that the implementation of community mental health services according to a "balanced care model" (see Chapters 1 and 10) is possible and desirable [13]. However, there is still a gap between population need and actual service provision across Europe, both between and within countries [11, 14]. To reduce the gap between the Eastern and Western parts of Europe and to scale up services across the region, the focus should be on the development of community-based services in the LAMICs, whilst sustaining and improving services in high-income settings. Furthermore, equal access for all needs to be ensured *within* countries; that is, across different regions and subgroups of the population [15,16]. Changes in service provision should be carefully planned to ensure gradual, balanced, and sustainable reform, which takes into account local conditions and resources, as well as the cultural context.

One important factor in making services accessible to whole populations is the continued integration of mental health services into primary health care, and an improvement in the quality of care within these systems. This may be facilitated by ensuring that there are sufficient numbers of primary care staff, regulating training, organizing adequate and ongoing supervision of primary care staff by mental health professionals, addressing staff attitudes, and developing and managing coordinated support networks with specialized community mental health services and other relevant sectors (such as social welfare, health, housing, and employment, as well as NGOs and the private sector) [17].

Human rights, stigma, and social inclusion

The lack of adequate community mental health services in many parts of Eastern Europe may often lead to the social isolation of people with mental health problems, or even a violation of their human rights through neglect and abuse [15]. Even in high-income countries (where community services tend to be more established) they may still be subject to stigma, prejudice, and discrimination [17]. National programs and plans should therefore be implemented to ensure that the human rights of people with mental disorders are upheld, their social inclusion and full integration into society (including in the workplace) is encouraged, and stigma and discrimination are reduced. These may include public mental health promotion, advocacy, and awareness-raising programs, both for the general population (for instance through media campaigns) as well as for health staff and personnel in the other relevant sectors mentioned above [15–17]. Furthermore, care services should be monitored and reviewed regularly to ensure that human rights standards are upheld [15]. Importantly, the views of service users, their families, and carers (as well as any other stakeholders) should be included in the planning and implementation of policies, and in service development, monitoring, and provision [2,13,15–17]. Currently, service user involvement is highest amongst EU-15 and other EU countries, but is only in the early stages of development in most Eastern European countries [15].

Legislation, policies, plans, and programs

One of the first steps in ensuring fair access to services for all is therefore the formulation of carefully planned mental health legislation and policies that take into account a wide range of stakeholders' views [16]. Even though there has been much progress in recent years, several countries in the European region still do not have adequate mental health legislation and policies in place. Comprehensive new national policies and legislation (including for the promotion, prevention, and advocacy of mental disorders) should be developed where these are absent, and older existing mental health policies and legislation should be updated. This needs to consist of a commitment not just by health ministries, but also by the other sectors already mentioned which may be relevant to mental health care [16, 17]. To address challenges in the implementation of these policies and to reduce the gap between mental health policy and practice, in particular in some of the Eastern and South-Eastern countries of the region [15], detailed, feasible (though ambitious), sustainable, and highly practical implementation plans and programs should be developed.

Resources (financial and human)

A common challenge in implementing mental health policies is the lack of adequate funding mechanisms for mental health, in particular in much of Eastern Europe [18]. Related to this is a shortage of human resources. Although mental health staff numbers have increased in many of the EU countries [16], with most of the mental health workforce in Europe being concentrated in a few high-income countries, human resources for mental health are still lacking in many other parts of Europe [15]; for example, whilst some of the high-income countries such as Belgium, Finland, and Iceland have over 20 psychiatrists per 100 000 population, other countries such as Tajikistan and Turkey have less than 2. This shortage typically results in mental institutions being retained and staff being assigned to mental institutions [17], which in turn leads to community mental health facilities being hugely understaffed [18]. Moreover, mental health workers are often underskilled due to insufficient resources for training [15, 17].

Since community mental health care overall has been shown to be cost-neutral compared to institutional care [2, 13, 19, 20], one solution in optimizing the use of available resources is to gradually shift financial and human resources from large mental institutions to community services [2, 13, 16, 19, 20]. This requires a changing of staff roles, responsibilities, and expertise, for instance through mental health workforce strategies [15], as well as new ongoing mental health training programs and an inclusion of mental health into general health care education programs [2, 13, 15–17]. Staff anxieties and uncertainties due to changing roles and service structures should also be addressed [2, 13], and working conditions and pathways for career development should be improved to reduce staff turnover [17].

Research evidence

An evidence base is vital to determine the effectiveness of community mental health services. However, this is still lacking for most countries in the European region, in particular outside the UK and other high-income (primarily EU-15) countries. High-quality and well-defined evaluative research is therefore needed across countries to strengthen the evidence base for clinical outcomes and cost-effectiveness of community mental health services, factors that may lead to their successful implementation and sustainability (in which service user-led research should be a focus), as well as the relative effectiveness and efficiency of policies and programs [15]. To avoid duplicating information unnecessarily, this should include standardizing data-collection systems and indicators across the region (for instance through the publishing of data-collection guidelines) [15–17] and forming a consensus on definitions of service components [15]. This, together with adequate dissemination systems, may enable evidence-based comparisons of services and programs to be made, which may in turn inform policies [15–17] and allow for a more informed allocation of limited resources [17].

North America

During five decades of developing community mental health programs in North America, several robust and durable concepts have emerged. These concepts contrast with many transient ideas that were never implemented broadly in real-world systems of care. The concepts correspond only loosely with research because research-based interventions sometimes fail to interest clients, providers, or payers. Some interventions take root and blossom over decades without much of a research base.

Team-based care

For people who have the most severe illnesses, the greatest disabilities, and the least amount of family or community support, integration of treatment, rehabilitation, and support services needs to be achieved at the clinical level [21]. Team-based care is the most straightforward way to ensure access, continuity, and integration of services. Teams make it possible to offer clients an individualized, coherent, and long-term program of medical, psychiatric, housing, financial, vocational, family, and social services to help them achieve their own goals. This insight emerged more than 30 years ago during early development of the assertive community treatment (ACT; see Appendix A) model and remains valid today.

Recovery

The recovery movement has spawned several important implications for the service delivery system: (i) it calls for widespread participation of peer-support workers within all types of service, and indeed, in the administration of and research on those services; (ii) it emphasizes choice and self-determination, so that the focus of services becomes helping clients achieve their own goals, as far as possible in their own way; (iii) it demands the replacement of unnecessarily coercive practices in favor of more clinically skilled, creative interactions within the context of mutually respectful, collaborative partnerships; and (iv) it also calls for funding consumer-run programs of various types that may have a weaker evidence base but that are favored by many people with mental illnesses.

Psychiatric rehabilitation and evidence-based practices

With its attention to the individual's goals, values, and preferences, the recovery movement has been consonant with parallel developments in the mental health field called psychiatric rehabilitation. One seminal paper described recovery as "the lived experience of rehabilitation" [22]. Within the rehabilitation movement, values (people first) and goals (successful adjustment in one's psychosocial areas of preference) have been consistent, methods and outcome measurements have evolved, and evidence-based practices have emerged [23]. Earlier stepwise approaches to rehabilitation based on lengthy psychotherapy and training programs have gradually been replaced by more modern approaches that involve helping clients to reach their goals rapidly by providing highly individualized support. Exemplars of the current approaches are supported housing, supported employment, supported education, and strengths case management.

Peer support

Social and instrumental support among peers with similar conditions has a long and robust history in North America. Alcoholics Anonymous, for example, has grown steadily since its development in the 1940s, and millions of people with alcoholism now attend Alcoholics Anonymous meetings in cities, suburbs, and towns throughout the region. Peer-support programs for people with severe and persistent mental disorders have proliferated for several decades [24]. Like Alcoholics Anonymous, they have been supported by the strong endorsement of people with these disorders themselves rather than by randomized controlled trials. Some 10–20% of people with severe mental disorders find these services helpful as a substitute for or an adjunct to community mental health services. The forms of peer services continue to evolve, but the concept has been enduring.

Economic consequences of neglect

In any mental health service system, a minority of individuals with mental illness consume a disproportionate share of expensive resources such as inpatient care, emergency room visits, incarcerations, and so on. Providing comprehensive, team-based care to these individuals is expensive, but it mitigates personal suffering, is no more costly, and avoids shifting the costs to families, communities, and the criminal justice system [25–27].

Implementation

As evidence-based practices have been defined with increasing precision and model fidelity, the inadequacy of brief training of frontline staff and team leaders has become clear. High-fidelity implementation requires ongoing training and supervision for six months to a year, and maintaining high-quality services also requires ongoing supervision [28–30].

The story of the development of community-based mental health services in the USA has been one of both hope and disappointment. It has been one of hope in that many of the most important innovations in the field have arisen there, from the most long-standing, extensive, and influential program of mental health services research in the world, as well as from a plethora of consumer initiatives; and also in that a few states have been trailblazers in showing how these advances can be turned into effective programs that actually help people with mental illnesses to recover. It has also been one of disappointment in that the political will and the funding levels needed to ensure development of these programs across the country have more often than not been lacking. Health care reform initiated by President Obama may change these trends.

Canada has imported many ideas from its neighbor to the south. While funding levels are more uniform than in the USA, and probably about adequate for good-quality care to be delivered throughout, various institutional arrangements, combined with lack of political will, have impeded the integration of state-of-the-art practices into routine care. Recent recognition of these failings by the federal government and the establishment of the Mental Health Commission of Canada may now lead to a period of accelerated progress.

Latin America and Caribbean

There are many lessons to be learned from the positive and negative experiences raised in developing community-based mental health care systems in Latin American and Caribbean countries. A summary of these lessons is given in Table 11.2. Most countries suffer from a scarcity of human resources, particularly psychiatrists and specialized nurses. Training nurses in Belize and mental health officers in Jamaica showed how effective these professionals were in treating severe psychiatric cases in the community. Another effective action was the training of general medical practitioners in Sobral, Brazil to care for psychiatric cases under close supervision of mental health professionals.

Reform means protecting the human rights of patients, being able to afford the best available treatments, treating severe cases in the community, and being as unrestrictive as possible. Denouncing abuse, human rights violations, and preventable deaths of people with mental disorders has also contributed to the closure of custodial hospitals in Brazil (Santos and Sobral) and Mexico. Moreover, the creation of specific laws protecting people with mental disorders and guaranteeing treatment was a triggering factor for boosting psychiatric reforms in Argentina, Brazil, and Mexico.

As demonstrated in Chile, it is possible to develop mental health programs at a national level on the basis of epidemiological studies and previously tested interventions by clinical trials. This Chilean initiative of using evidence-based data and the burden of mental disorders to design a

Table 11.2 Lessons learned in overcoming barriers in the implementation of community mental health services in some of the Latin American and Caribbean countries.

Country	Lessons learned
Argentina	• Having local community mental health care in the region has led to a decrease of 80% of the referral of users to mental health services outside of province [57]. • Training and showing positive results have been important in reducing resistance and helping doctors better manage patients with mental disorders [3]. • Training in mental health and primary care for residents have been important for the integration of mental health into primary care [57]. • A high level of political commitment has contributed to the success of the Austral program in Neuquén [3].
Belize	• Psychiatric nurses can increase awareness of mental health issues, in health sectors and in others. • Systematic mental health training for general practitioners and community nurses is crucial to maintaining quality of care [3]. • Low salaries are an important constraint to retaining mental health professionals in the system (brain-drain) [58]. • The National Mental Health Plan is a cornerstone for implementing and improving access and service quality. • Legislation to protect the rights of people with mental disabilities is an important factor for boosting psychiatric reform [58].
Brazil	• Regular and close supervision in mental health for health teams in primary care (nurses and general practitioners) are essential for avoiding unnecessary patient referral to mental health specialists and for quality of care [3, 59]. • Extensive and regular training of nurses in mental health is essential. • Improvement of the collection and monitoring of data is important to establishing communication between primary and secondary care, and to evaluating efficiency of services [60]. • Decreasing bureaucratic constraints (between municipalities, federal government, and states), and revising incompatibilities between national and regional laws, is crucial to facilitating service implementation and functioning [61].
Chile	• In setting up priorities, by using DALYs to measure burden of disease, it has been important to have solid previous epidemiological data showing the importance of depression among lower-class women and alcohol dependence among men [62–66]. • The number of people attending the victims of the dictatorship program only increased after Britain took legal action against Pinochet [67]. • Services have been set up within an established geographical area, looking for integration and a common coordination [67]. • There was resistance to the acceptance of a new set of priorities and new organization of services. Different components found it hard to work together as a team, and there was a difficult period of integration [67].
Cuba	• The Cuban mental health system has strong bases for primary care, decentralization, and community participation, with a strong family doctor system covering the whole population [68].

Table 11.2 Continued.

Country	Lessons learned
	• Good public education about mental disorders contributes to strong participation and political power inside the country [68].
	• Trained personnel at the primary care level and a strong and constant mental health network guarantee the efficacy of this system [69].
Jamaica	• Mental health officers (MHOs) are trained quicker and offer a community service unlikely to be fulfilled by doctors. MHOs may represent a cost-effective strategy to meet community care needs in regions where there are insufficient doctors [70].
	• A mental health act allows MHOs to practice detention [71].
Mexico	• NGOs (MDRI and FMREM) and civilian activists have played a crucial role in triggering the reform process by denouncing extreme situations and human rights violations in psychiatric institutions, and have brought about mental health reform in cooperation with the Ministry of Health [72].

mental health plan should be followed, especially by those countries with more financial resources like Brazil, Argentina, and Mexico.

The main ingredients to guide mental health policies should be public health needs, human rights protection, and cost-effective and evidence-based interventions. Another important step is to monitor changes by using health indicators to evaluate actions, as in Belize, so as to assess the efficiency and effectiveness of services.

It is necessary to have a budget for mental health. There are many examples in Latin American and Caribbean countries of the lack of financial resources even for basic needs such as fuel, transportation, telephone calls, and provision of medicines. A good mental health plan should encompass the financial resources required for an efficient care delivery; most countries in the region spend less than 1% of the total health budget on mental health.

Partnership with NGOs, private institutions, and other international agencies was effective in triggering psychiatric reform in Mexico (Hidalgo experience) through the advocacy of the human rights of people with mental disorders. Furthermore, an NGO partnership was seen in Argentina (Neuquén), through the Austral program, which included training of mental health professionals and provided rehabilitation for people with mental disorders. The participation of NGOs in Latin American and Caribbean countries can be considered modest when compared to their roles in Asia and Africa.

It is noteworthy that, in some cases, psychiatric beds have been closed without a concomitant development of community resources. No mental health system can function with insufficient beds for acute admissions [31]. Experiences in which there were fewer acute beds than needed, as in the Santos case, led to the transference of acute cases to other cities, causing unnecessary pain and suffering to patients and their families. Therefore, psychiatric beds should only be removed where there is an adequate community infrastructure in place to take care of patients and families.

This review has shown that custodial care is in the process of being abolished in Latin American and Caribbean countries: mental health is now integrated more into primary care and many acute-episode patients have been treated in psychiatric wards of general hospitals. However, the composite picture describing progress in the region includes the recognition that few community-based services are available, particularly for children and adolescents, and that the capacity to monitor and evaluate services and programs remains insufficient. The current reality of very small budgets for mental health in most countries leads to an array of failures in the system: insufficient supplies of medicines, few residential facilities for the mentally ill, and an overload of work for low-paid mental health professionals.

In South America and the Caribbean, custodial care is in the process of being abolished, and mental health is now more integrated into primary care. Many acute psychiatric episodes are now being treated in the psychiatric wards of general hospitals. Despite the progress seen in the region, many steps must still be taken to reduce the burden of mental disorders: lack of specialized professionals, shortage of community mental health centers—particularly for children—, absence of mental health legislation and planning, low budgets for mental health, insufficient supplies of medicines, few residential facilities for the mentally ill, and an overload of work for mental health professionals.

South Asia

Policy and planning

Many policy makers are oblivious to the importance of mental health. Mental health is not a priority area for many governments in this region and hence the funds allocated are quite meager. The absence of a national plan or policy for community mental health in many countries of the region has also contributed to the low priority accorded to community-based programs. Funding nationally and internationally does not come easily for community mental health projects.

This situation is however changing, at least in India. The 10th five-year plan has increased the allocation of funds to mental health, although a bulk of it will be spent on improving the conditions of mental hospitals. A portion has also been allocated to district mental health programs in various states.

Professional challenges

A huge brain-drain has left some of the countries in the region with much fewer psychiatrists. There is also a lack of other mental health professionals, such as clinical psychologists, social workers, and psychiatric nurses. The governments of these countries should work out methods to reduce this outflow of trained professionals.

In the absence of required numbers of trained professionals, there arises a need to involve community-level health workers, teachers, volunteers, key persons in the local community, and family members, in the process of identifying persons with mental disorders, making appropriate referrals, and providing care and simple psychosocial interventions. This has been successfully done in Sri Lanka, where Community Support Officers (CSOs), a new cadre of mental health workers, were established in the wake of the tsunami, after it was evident that in most tsunami districts the basic primary care services were overwhelmed and could not take on any additional activities [32].

This should be confined, at least initially, to a few major mental health conditions such as psychoses, depression, substance abuse and so on, rather than expose them to a wide gamut of overlapping conditions. The chosen psychosocial interventions also need to be simple and largely targeted at economic activities.

Training and capacity building are also critical pieces of the puzzle and should form an integral part of all community-oriented activities. This would necessitate the use of simple information technologies, periodic re-inforcer sessions, and a component of evaluation.

Existing primary care physicians in the community are not always ready or inclined to treat the mentally ill. Whilst training them enhances their skills, they should be sufficiently motivated to take on the additional responsibility of caring for the mentally ill. Innovations to beat the challenge of inadequate personnel include the use of telepsychiatry, which is being successfully employed in Tamil Nadu, a Southern Indian state, by the NGO Schizophrenia Research Foundation [33].

Population challenges

For centuries, communities in the region have held competing explanatory magico-religious models to understand and explain mental illness in the least stigmatizing way possible. This in turn results in the use of traditional and religious modes of care, which often causes considerable delay in seeking medical help. Demystifying and simplifying mental disorders in a manner understood and accepted by the local community is another challenge.

Development of mental health services should take into account local needs and requirements—community consultation should be the starting point. The challenge is not only to be culturally and socially sensitive, but also to integrate local expertise and systems of medicine such as Ayurveda or Siddha with Western medical practices.

Recommendations for the South Asia region

Increase the mental health budget

Reallocation of the mental health budget is called for in many countries in the region, since a large part of the budget is spent on mental hospitals which house long-stay patients with minimal turnover. There needs to be an increased allocation for community-based care and to help families cope with the problem.

Increase access for patients

One of the pitfalls of community-based programs, particularly in rural areas, is the lack of access to these services. The evaluation report of the district mental health program in India recommended strengthening "services at sub-centers, and Primary Health Centre level so that the services become more accessible to the patients". Unless community systems of care are strengthened, many patients will continue to be untreated.

Capacity building

Community care requires a balanced mix of clinical skills and practical knowledge of working in and with communities. Continuing professional development in the form of continuing medical education (CME), and equipping professionals with skills based on evidence, is critical. In many areas in this region, this translates into a greater emphasis on mental health at the undergraduate level. Special programs for immigrants, during and after disasters, and for the socially and economically marginalized—such as poor women or children (especially in rural areas)—need to be drawn up and the required training imparted. Some countries, such as India, have drawn up clinical and practice guidelines which need to be disseminated widely to provide uniformity in care.

For the system to be culturally and locally relevant, it is useful to understand people's perception of mental health needs. In 2008, a training workshop was held in Sri Lanka in collaboration with McGill University in Canada to provide participants with a better understanding of local communities. Fernando et al. [34] suggest three overlapping stages:

1 Dialogue and consultation with communities.
2 Capacity building with local mental health workers.
3 Integration of the system into social welfare and health structures.

In the absence of qualified mental health professionals, many countries have trained lay community workers, as in the case of community support officers in Sri Lanka. These community support officers have significantly enhanced both the overall access to and coverage of mental health services to communities across all four districts, particularly in areas where there was previously limited or no local access to psychiatric care (either due to protracted civil conflict or lack of mental health service structures) [32].

For the training of lay community workers, several organizations have developed tool kits and manuals in local languages, and these should also be disseminated widely and put to use.

Strong action for mental health awareness and stigma reduction

There should be mass publicity of awareness programs through local media—print, audio (community radio), and visual (local TV channels)—as well as camps/classes in schools, colleges, and other educational institutions. There is a felt need for promotive components such as suicide prevention, workplace stress management, and school and college counseling services, as well as an integration/coordination of mental health programs with other health programs, such as those for women and children, or rural development.

Community mental health services in this region should be evidence-based, yet be receptive and responsive to the needs of local communities. A strong psychosocial approach should exist alongside the biomedical approach currently practiced. Priority should be given to the needs of rural areas—since most of the population in these countries lives in villages—, essential medicines, and support and supervision of health personnel.

East and South-East Asia

Obstacles and challenges in East and South-East Asia

Human rights

Traditional beliefs that mental illnesses are caused by malicious spirit possession or weak character persist. According to a national survey in South Korea, people often consider mental illnesses to be self-limiting disorders that will resolve on their own [35]. Much stigma is still attached to persons with mental illness, as well as to psychiatric institutions and services. Some people avoid such services because of these negative images [36]. One study found that the major predictors of people seeking help are not availability and access to care, but rather health beliefs about perceptions of mental illness and health care [37]. Public misconceptions about mental illness result in prejudice which in turn leads to discrimination. There is a gap between legal frameworks and the reality of the mentally ill, who are often abused in many countries [38].

Family involvement

Strong family involvement in mental health care and treatment is characteristic of Asia. Family plays an essential role in the care of people with mental disorders in the community; however, poor knowledge of mental illness and negative attitudes about the patient prevent many people in need from seeking care [39]. Many persons with mental illness are abandoned by their families. The establishment of partnerships with families and the assignment of necessary resources are challenges in this field of patient care.

Traditional healers

In many countries in the region, it is common for people to consult traditional healers from complementary and alternative medicine for their health problems, even if medical services are available. Healers rarely cooperate with each other, nor do they collectively work with formal health care providers [40]. Cambodians often seek help from Kru Khmers, who are mainly herbalists [41], and it is also common to consult traditional healers in East-Timor [42]. Families often bring the patient to religious healers first, although the government of Vietnam prohibits this act [43]. In Indonesia, up to 80% of people consult traditional healers as a first resort [44]. A 1993 survey in Singapore showed that 30% of patients in a national hospital visited traditional healers, *dukun*, before consulting physicians [45]. Such behavior is one of the reasons for the low formal service use in the region.

Distribution of service provision/continuity of care

Mental health services are available only in certain areas of countries. Most people with severe mental disorders are unable to access services in low-resource countries, and mental health resources are centralized in large cities in medium-resource countries.

A gradual transition from psychiatric hospitals to community care has occurred, and the recent focus in most countries in the region has been on shortening the length of stay. Intensive community care, crisis intervention, and an urgent referral system are crucial for patients after discharge, though seamless care is not easy. In Japan and South Korea, policy proposals exist to convert current long-term psychiatric care beds to outpatient/ambulatory clinics or long-term community-based care, but in reality many discharged patients have failed to make use of such services. A survey in South Korea showed a high readmission rate immediately after discharge [46], whilst one in Malaysia reported a lower rate of followed-up and treated patients at one year [47]. South Korea is quickly developing a comprehensive mental health service system in each catchment area [48].

In Japan, people lack an awareness of the "catchment area" due to the negative effects of the universal insurance system, which is the greatest contribution to Japanese health [49].

Financial resources

Most of the countries in the region are seeking to balance public and private financing and provision of care. The source of funds for the development of community services is usually savings made from the reduction of beds in hospitals, though such cutbacks and increasing community services are not always balanced. Furthermore, in rapidly aging countries, community services are urgently needed for people with dementia. There is concern that most of the mental health budgets will be spent on treating those with this disease. If the boundary between mental health and elderly care becomes unclear, a smaller amount of money will be earmarked for people with severe and persistent mental disorders.

Lessons learned and recommendations in East and South-East Asia

Legal processes and anti-stigma campaigns

Legal processes are needed to protect the human rights of persons with mental illnesses in countries where appropriate legislation is absent. In Japan, the Mental Health Act legally acknowledges for the first time that mental illness is a disability, and stricter criteria and a Psychiatric Review Board for involuntary admissions have been established after a series of scandals regarding human rights violations [50].

In the context of anti-stigma campaigns, renaming a disease is generally well accepted in Japan and Hong Kong [51, 52]. Similar movements are seen in other East Asian countries where Chinese characters are used.

Integration with the general health system

Even with minimal resources, the simple creation of an accessible service makes a difference [53]. The best way to create a cost-effective system is to utilize the existing general medical sector, including training of primary health workers. Singapore has been successful in preparing general practitioners for treating, with psychiatrists' support, patients with mental illness [54].

Better access to mental health services is available at the primary care level because it is closer to home, and primary care is generally more acceptable to persons with mental disorders and their families. Not much embarrassment or stigma is encountered by help-seekers in the primary mental health services [54]. Collaborative networks are needed among stakeholders to avoid fragmentation and must include service users/families, hospitals, community health workers, NGOs, and traditional healers.

Prioritization of target groups

Due to limited resources, care needs to be prioritized. Compared to depression or mild mental disorders, which are generally more accepted and better funded, persons with severe and persistent mental disorders are often omitted and left behind in planning and budgeting. Prioritized services should be provided to severely disabled persons.

Leadership and policy making

Strong leadership is needed to navigate changes. Very few mental health professionals are actively involved in policy making. Consequently, the lack of leadership allows the allocation of more money or resources to general health care services rather than to mental health. It is not uncommon for non-mental health professionals to have negative attitudes towards mental illness. It is therefore necessary to change their ways of thinking.

Not only central but also local governments need to participate in the development of sustainable community mental health care systems. In recent times, former patients, "survivors", have had more opportunities to speak publicly and participate in mental health policy making [55].

Funds and economic incentives

First, overall mental health budgets should be increased. Persons with mental illness often suffer from unemployment and subsequent poverty; therefore, out-of-pocket funds are needed for mental health care. This financial insecurity keeps persons with mental illness and their families from seeking medical services. It is essential to develop a funding system in which all people who need help are able to receive it.

Economic incentives are necessary to promote community-based mental care services. Hospitals and mental health professionals are reluctant to shift to the community because of poorer funding and lower salaries [56]. One of the ideas is to reduce inpatient payments and to increase community service fees. However, caution is needed because some long-stay patients are often severely disabled or old; alternative care may be needed for such patients. Transitional costs may be necessary for retraining of mental health workers. ACT and employment support are not fully covered by medical expenditures. A flexible financial structure over medical and social boundaries is therefore required.

After a long history of resorting to asylum, a slow deinstitutionalization is occurring in East and South-East Asia, and this region is now in a transition period from institutional to community care. Unlike the West, Asian countries fear the confusion engendered by rapid change; they are cautiously reducing or closing psychiatric hospitals, and simultaneously trying to build community services. This attempt has not yet been successful, mainly because of system fragmentation. Role differentiation is required between hospitals and community services, and public and private services. Ensuring quality of care is the next challenge for community mental health care. We can learn lessons from other regions in constructing the future of mental health care in East and South-East Asia.

This book has brought together a wealth of information, both from the literature and from hard-won experience on the ground, on how to conceive and deliver better mental health care. As these pages show, the challenges are formidable, and therefore our determination must be at least as great. From the many examples across all the chapters, it is clear that services can best develop if guided clearly by: (i) a principled ethical base (paying particular attention to the observation of human rights of people with mental illness); (ii) the evidential base (learning from the research literature which services and treatments are effective and cost-effective); and (iii) the experiential base (the accumulated experience of both those providing services and those with mental illness, their carers and their family members (the intended beneficiaries) about which approaches have been found, through trial and error, to lead to better mental health care).

Key points in this chapter

- Key mistakes in implementing community mental health care across regions worldwide include a lack of a carefully considered sequence of events linking hospital bed closure to community service development, attempting system reform without including *all* the relevant stakeholders, linking inappropriately the reform of mental health care with narrow ideological or party-political interests, an exclusive focus of community services on psychotic conditions, and the neglect of patients' physical health.
- Obstacles, challenges, lessons learned, and solutions in the implementation of community mental health care worldwide include those relating to:
  - Society (for instance the disregard or violation of human rights, as well as stigma and discrimination).
  - Government (for example the low priority given to mental health, inadequate mental health policies or legislation, or insufficient financial resources).
  - The organization of the local mental health system (for instance the lack of mental health programs, the poor use of mental health facilities, or the lack of multisectoral collaboration).

- ○ Professionals and practitioners (for example the need for leadership, inadequate training and supervision, or high staff turnover and burnout).
  - ○ Users, families, and other advocates (for instance the need for advocacy, self-help, or shared decision making).
- Services can best develop if guided clearly by a principled ethical base, evidential base, and experiential base.
- For the Africa region, challenges in the implementation of community mental health care include competing priorities, waning community engagement, reliance on community volunteers not being sustainable, under-funding, the paucity of mental health professionals, negative attitudes to mental health, concern about skills of staff and quality of care, difficulty sustaining in-service training, erratic supplies of psychotropic medication, lack of multisectoral collaboration (including traditional healers), and an escalating need and demand for services. Lessons learned for the region include that it can be done, the need for patience, perseverance and determination, that sustainability requires making best use of existing systems, the need to identify and cultivate allies for support, that advocacy and community groups can influence policy makers, that supervision of primary health care workers is necessary, the importance of proper planning, the need to integrate evaluation and monitoring, and that the marginalization of mental health can block progress. Recommendations for the region include the strengthening of specialist mental health services whilst simultaneously integrating mental health into primary health care, increasing the quality and sustainability of mental health in primary health care through adequate supervision, ongoing on-the-job training and reliable referral networks, developing robust mechanisms to ensure reliable supplies of psychotropic medications, supporting the provision of simple and feasible psychosocial interventions to augment medication approaches in the time-pressed primary health care setting, and conducting evaluative research.
- In Australia and New Zealand, lessons learned about what is required for the change process to succeed include the importance of a sustained incremental approach over decades, cross-party support, funding that is "ring-fenced", planning that is accompanied by costed and scheduled implementation plans and mechanisms to hold agencies accountable for achieving results, service champions as leaders of change, understanding the specificities of local communities and how to engage community support, expertise in and commitment to models of collaborative care, broad-based coalitions leading to a mandated process of transparent consultation, a strong and varied workforce, and service evaluation and quality improvement. In the Pacific Nations, lessons learned include the importance of governments being encouraged to develop national

policies and plans to address the needs of those with serious mental illnesses based on models of community care, the need for this to occur in tandem with educational efforts to increase local people's knowledge of mental illness and what can be done to help family members who have developed mental illnesses, educational opportunities for general health professionals to gain and upskill their knowledge and practice in the recognition and treatment of mental illness, enabling visiting specialist mental health professionals to provide consultation-liaison support for generally trained health professionals, acknowledging and engaging the input of traditional healers and family members, and encouraging the development of mental health care pathways and referral systems.

- In the Europe region, lessons learned and recommendations for the implementation of community mental health care relate to a reduction in the treatment gap between population need and actual service provision, a lessening of human rights abuses, stigma and social exclusion, the development of adequate legislation, policies, plans and programs, an increase in financial and human resources, and the strengthening of research evidence.
- In North America, robust and durable concepts for community mental health care that have emerged include team-based care, the recovery movement, psychiatric rehabilitation and evidence-based practices, peer support, issues related to the economic consequences of neglect, and the importance of high-fidelity implementation.
- In the Latin America and Caribbean region, there is currently a lack of specialized professionals, a shortage of community mental health centers, an absence of mental health legislation and planning, a low budget for mental health, insufficient supplies of medicines, few residential facilities for the mentally ill, and an overload of work for mental health professionals. Lessons learned in the implementation of community mental health care include that it is possible to develop mental health programs at a national level, the need for a focus on public health needs, human rights protection and cost-effective and evidence-based interventions, the need for a mental health budget, and the benefits of partnerships between agencies and organizations.
- In the South Asia region, challenges in the implementation of community health care relate to policy and planning (for instance the lack of national mental health plans or policies), professional challenges (such as brain-drain), and population challenges (for example delays in help seeking due to explanatory magico-religious models). Recommendations for the region include an increase in the mental health budget, increasing access to patients, capacity building, and the need for strong action for mental health awareness and stigma reduction.
- In the East and South-East Asia region, obstacles and challenges in the implementation of community mental health care include abuses of

human rights, strong family involvements, a large presence of traditional healers, an unequal distribution in service provision and continuity of care, and the scarcity of financial resources. Lessons learned and recommendations for the region include the need for legal processes and anti-stigma campaigns, integration with the general health system, the prioritization of target groups, the need for strong leadership and policy making, and the need for more funds and economic incentives.

References

[1] Saraceno B, van Ommeren M, Batniji R, Cohen A, Gureje O, Mahoney J, et al. Barriers to improvement of mental health services in low-income and middle-income countries. Lancet 2007;370:1164–74.

[2] Thornicroft G, Tansella M, Law A. Steps, challenges and lessons in developing community mental health care. World Psychiatry 2008;7:87–92.

[3] World Health Organization and Wonca. Integrating Mental Health into Primary Care: A Global Perspective. Geneva: WHO and World Organization of Family Doctors; 2008.

[4] Kigozi F. Integrating mental health into primary health care—Uganda's experience. African Journal of Psychiatry 2007;10:17–19.

[5] BasicNeeds. Community Mental Health Practice: Seven Essential Features for Scaling Up in Low- and Middle-Income Countries. Bangalore; 2009.

[6] Ben-Tovim DI. A psychiatric service to the remote areas of Botswana. British Journal of Psychiatry 1983;142:199–203.

[7] Ben-Tovim DI, Kundu P. Botswana: Integration of psychiatric care with primary health care. Lancet 1982;320(8301):757–8.

[8] Cohen A. The Effectiveness of Mental Health Services in Primary Care: The View from the Developing World. Geneva: WHO; 2001.

[9] Swartz L, MacGregor H. Integrating services, marginalizing patients: Psychiatric patients and primary health care in South Africa. Transcultural Psychiatry 2002;39(2):155–72.

[10] Lancet Global Mental Health Group. Global mental health. 6. Scale up services for mental disorders: A call for action. Lancet 2007;370:87–98.

[11] World Health Organization. Mental Health Gap Action Programme—Scaling Up Care for Mental, Neurological, and Substance Use Disorders. Geneva: WHO; 2008.

[12] Sartorius N, Harding TW. The WHO collaborative study on strategies for extending mental health care. I. The genesis of the study. Geneva: WHO; 1983.

[13] Thornicroft G, Tansella M. Better Mental Health Care. Cambridge: Cambridge University Press; 2009.

[14] World Health Organization. Mental Health Services in Europe: The Treatment Gap Briefing Paper, WHO European Ministerial Conference on Mental Health, Helsinki, 12–15 January 2005. WHO; 2005.

[15] World Health Organization. Policies and Practices for Mental Health in Europe—Meeting the Challenges. Geneva: WHO; 2008.

[16] European Commission. The State of Mental Health in the European Union. European Commission; 2004.

[17] World Health Organization. Mental Health: Facing the Challenges, Building Solutions—Report from the WHO European Ministerial Conference. Copenhagen: WHO Regional Office for Europe; 2005.

[18] Knapp M, McDaid D, Mossialos E, Thornicroft G. Mental health policy and practice across Europe: An overview. In: Knapp M, McDaid D, Mossialos E, Thornicroft G, editors. Mental Health Policy and Practice across Europe. Maidenhead: Open University Press; 2007. pp. 1–14.

[19] Thornicroft G, Tansella M. What are the Arguments for Community-Based Mental Health Care? Copenhagen: WHO Regional Office for Europe; 2003.

[20] Thornicroft G, Tansella M. Components of a modern mental health service: A pragmatic balance of community and hospital care—Overview of systematic evidence. British Journal of Psychiatry 2004;185:283–90.

[21] Lehman A, Kreyenbuhl J, Buchanan R, Dickerson FB, Dixon LB, Goldberg R, et al. The schizophrenia patient outcomes research team (PORT): Updated treatment recommendations 2003. Schizophrenia Bulletin 2004;30:193–217.

[22] Deegan P. Recovery: The lived experience of rehabilitation. Psychosocial Rehabilitation 1988;11:11–19.

[23] Turner J, TenHoor W. The NIMH community support program: Pilot approach to a needed social reform. Schizophrenia Bulletin 1978;4:319–48.

[24] Solomon P. Peer support/peer provided services underlying processes, benefits, and critical ingredients. Psychiatric Rehabilitation Journal 2004;27:392–401.

[25] Culhane D. The costs of homelessness: A perspective from the United States. European Journal of Homelessness 2008;2:97–114.

[26] Larimer M, Malone D, Garner M, Atkins DC, Burlingham B, Lonczak HS, et al. Health care and public service use and costs before and after provision of housing for chronically homeless persons with severe alcohol problems. JAMA 2009;301:1349–57.

[27] Latimer E. Economic impacts of assertive community treatment: A review of the literature. Canadian Journal of Psychiatry 1999;44:443–54.

[28] Drake R, Bond G, Essock S. Implementing evidence-based practices for people with schizophrenia. Schizophrenia Bulletin 2009;35:704–13.

[29] Fixsen D, Naoom SF, Blase KA, Friedman RM, Wallace F. Implementation Research: A Synthesis of the Literature. Tampa: University of South Florida; 2005.

[30] Rapp C, Etzel-Wise D, Marty D, Coffman M, Carlson L, Asher D, et al. Evidence-based practice implementation strategies: Results of a qualitative study. Community Mental Health Journal 2008;44:213–24.

[31] Thornicroft G, Alem A, Antunes Dos Santos R, Barley E, Drake RE, Gregorio G, et al. WPA guidance on steps, obstacles and mistakes to avoid in the implementation of community mental health care. World Psychiatry 2010;9:67–77.

[32] Wickramage K, Suveendran T, Mahoney J. Mental Health in Sri Lanka—Evaluation of the Impact of Community Support Officers (CSO) in Mental Health Service Provision at District Level. Colombo: WHO Country Office; 2009.

[33] Thara R, Islam A, Padmavati R. Beliefs about mental illness: A study of a rural South Indian Community. International Journal of Mental Health 1998;27: 70–85.

[34] Fernando S, Weerackody C. Challenges in developing community mental health services in Sri Lanka. J of Health Management 2009;11(1):195–208.

[35] Cho SJ, Lee JY, Hong JP, Lee HB, Cho MJ, Hahm BJ. Mental health service use in a nationwide sample of Korean adults. Social Psychiatry & Psychiatric Epidemiology 2009;44:943–51.

[36] Wei KC, Lee C, Wong KE. Community psychiatry in Singapore: An integration of community mental health services towards better patient care. The Hong Kong Journal of Psychiatry 2005;15:132–7.

[37] Ng TP, Jun AZ, Ho R, Chua HC, Fones CS, Lim L. Health beliefs and help seeking for depressive and anxiety disorders among urban Singaporean adults. Psychiatric Services, 2008;59:105–8.

[38] Irmansyah I, Prasetyo YA, Minas H. Human rights of persons with mental illness in Indonesia: More than legislation is needed. International Journal of Mental Health Systems 2009;3:14.

[39] Phillips MR, Zhang J, Shi Q, Song Z, Ding Z, Pang S, et al. Prevalence, treatment, and associated disability of mental disorders in four provinces in China during 2001–05: An epidemiological survey. Lancet 2009;373:2041–53.

[40] Parameshvara DM. Malaysia mental health country profile. International Review of Psychiatry 2004;16:167–76.

[41] Collins W. Medical Practitioners and Traditional Healers: A Study of Health Seeking Behavior in Kampong Chhnang, Cambodia. Phnom Penh, Cambodia: Health Economics Task Force, Ministry of Health, The Provincial Health Department, Kampong Chhnang and the WHO Health Sector Reform Project Team; 2000.

[42] Zwi AB, Silove D. Hearing the voices: Mental health services in East-Timor. Lancet 2002;360:S45–6.

[43] Uemoto M. Viet Nam. In: Shinfuku N, Asai K, editors. Mental Health in the World, revised edition. Tokyo: Health Press; 2009. pp. 107–11.

[44] Pols H. The development of psychiatry in Indonesia: From colonial to modern times. International Review of Psychiatry 2006;18:363–70.

[45] Yoshida N. ASEAN countries. In: Shinfuku N, Asai K, editors. Mental Health in the World, revised edition. Tokyo: Health Press; 2009.

[46] Lee MS, Hoe M, Hwang TY, Lee YM. Service priority and standard performance of community mental health centers in South Korea: A Delphi approach. Psychiatry Investigation 2009;6:59–65.

[47] Salleh MR. Decentralization of psychiatric services in Malaysia: What is the prospect? Singapore Medical Journal 1993;34:139–41.

[48] World Health Organization. WHO-AIMS Report on Mental Health System in Republic of Korea. Gwacheon City, Republic of Korea: WHO and Ministry of Health and Welfare; 2007.

[49] Ito H. Quality and performance improvement for mental healthcare in Japan. Current Opinion in Psychiatry 2009;22:619–22.

[50] Ito H, Sederer LI. Mental health services reform in Japan. Harvard Review of Psychiatry 1999;7:208–15.

[51] Chen E, Chen C. The impact of renamed schizophrenia in psychiatric practice in Hong Kong. In: The Second World Congress of Asian Psychiatry, 7–10th November, 2009. Taipei, Taiwan; 2009.

[52] Sato M. Renaming schizophrenia: A Japanese perspective. World Psychiatry 2006;5:53–5.

[53] Jones L, Asare JB, Masri ME, Mohanraj A, Sherief H, van Ommeren M. Severe mental disorders in complex emergencies. Lancet 2009;374:654–61.

[54] Lum AW, Kwok KW, Chong SA. Providing integrated mental health services in the Singapore primary care setting—The general practitioner psychiatric programme experience. ANNALS Academy of Medicine Singapore 2008;37:128–31.

[55] Kuno E, Asukai N. Efforts toward building a community-based mental health system in Japan. International Journal of Law and Psychiatry 2000;23:361–73.

[56] Phillips MR. Mental health services in China. Epidemiologia e Psichiatria Sociale 2000;9:84–8.

[57] Collins PY. Argentina: Waving the mental health revolution banner—Psychiatric reform and community mental health in the province of Rio Negro. In: Ameida JMC, Cohen A, editors. Innovative Mental Health Programs in Latin America and the Caribbean. Washington: Pan American Health Organization (PAHO); 2008. pp. 1–32.

[58] Killion C, Cayetano C. Making mental health a priority in Belize. Archives of Psychiatric Nursing 2009;23:157–65.

[59] Silveira MR, Alves M. O enfermeiro na equipe de saúde mental—O caso dos CERSAMs de Belo Horizonte. Revista Latino-americana de Enfermagem 2003;11:645–51.

[60] Oliveira GL, Caiaffa WT, Cherchiglia ML. [Mental health and continuity of care in healthcare centers in a city of Southeastern Brazil]. Revista Panamericana de Salud Pública 2008;42:707–16.

[61] Furtado JP. [Needs evaluation of the Sheltered Homes in Brazilian public health system]. Ciência & saúde coletiva 2006;11:785–95.

[62] Araya R, Rojas G, Fritsch R, Acuna J, Lewis G. Common mental disorders in Santiago, Chile: Prevalence and socio-demographic correlates. The British Journal of Psychiatry 2001;178:228–33.

[63] Araya R, Wynn R, Leonard R, Lewis G. Psychiatric morbidity in primary health care in Santiago, Chile: Preliminary findings. The British Journal of Psychiatry 1994;165:530–3.

[64] Minoletti A, López C. Las enfermedades mentales en Chile: Magnitud y consecuencias. Santiago: Ministerio de Salud; 1999.

[65] Vicente B, Kohn R, Rioseco P, Saldivia S, Levav I, Torres S. Lifetime and 12-month prevalence of DSM-III-R disorders in the Chile psychiatric prevalence study. American Journal of Psychiatry, 2006;163:1362–70.

[66] Vicente B, Rioseco P, Saldivia S, Kohn R, Torres S. [Chilean study on the prevalence of psychiatric disorders (DSM-III-R/CIDI) (ECPP)]. Revista Médica de Chile 2002;130:527–36.

[67] Frammer CM. Chile: Reforms in national mental health policy. In: Almeida JM, Cohen A, editors. Innovative Mental Health Programs in Latin America and the Caribbean. Washington: Pan American Health Organization (PAHO); 2008. pp. 44–60.

[68] Basauri VA. Cuba: Mental health care and community participation. In: Almeida JM, Cohen A, editors. Innovative Mental Health Programs in Latin America and the Caribbean. Washington: Pan American Health Organization (PAHO); 2008. pp. 67–79.

[69] Hernandez BJ, Cabeza AA, Lopez F. La reorientación de la salud mental hacia la atención primaria en la provincia de Cienfuegos: Departamento de Salud Mental de la Provincia de Cienfuegos. In: Hernandez BJ, Cabeza AA, Lopez F, editors. Enfoques para um debate en salud mental. Havana: Ediciones Conexiones; 2002. pp. 109–37.

[70] McKenzie, K. Jamaica: Community mental health services. In: Almeida JM, Cohen A, editors. Innovative Mental Health Programs in Latin America and the Caribbean. Washington: Pan American Health Organization (PAHO); 2008. pp. 79–92.

[71] Jamaica. Mental Health Act 1997. Jamaica: Government Printing Services; 1997.

[72] Xavier M. Mexico: The Hidalgo experience—A new approach to mental health care. In: Almeida JM, Cohen A, editors. Innovative Mental Health Programs in Latin America and the Caribbean. Washington: Pan American Health Organization (PAHO); 2008. pp. 97–111.

APPENDIX A
Terminologies

People with mental disorders

A wide range of terms are used to describe people with mental disorders worldwide, including "patients", "service users", "users", "clients", "consumers", and "survivors". Similarly, a wide range of terms may be used worldwide to describe different disorders. Even though standard terminologies used may vary across different countries, it is important to be respectful when describing people with mental disorders, in accordance with countries' cultural beliefs and norms. We have tried to use terminologies that are appropriate cross-culturally (as far as is possible) throughout this book.

Overview and definitions of community mental health services

A range of services have been developed which enable the client to be treated in the community rather than in hospital. Most have been developed within Europe and North America, where they can be considered to fall into three levels of care: primary care, general adult mental health care, and specialized services.

General adult mental health services include: acute inpatient care, community mental health teams (CMHTs), long-term community-based residential care, outpatient/ambulatory clinics, and work and occupation.

Specialized services include: alternatives to acute inpatient care (including acute day hospitals, crisis houses, and home-treatment/crisis-resolution teams), specialized CMHTs (including assertive community treatment (ACT) teams and early-intervention teams), alternative types of long-stay community residential care (including 24-hour staffed residential care, day-staffed residential facilities, and lower supported accommodation), specialized outpatient/ambulatory clinics, and specialized forms of work and occupation.

Community Mental Health: putting policy into practice globally, First Edition. Graham Thornicroft, Maya Semrau, Atalay Alem, Robert E. Drake, Hiroto Ito, Jair Mari, Peter McGeorge, and R. Thara. © 2011 John Wiley & Sons, Ltd. Published 2011 by John Wiley & Sons, Ltd.

Primary care mental health services

Three models of care have been developed to improve mental health care within a primary care setting: "collaborative care", "consultation liaison", and "replacement" [1].

The collaborative care model

This is an enhanced form of consultation liaison which also includes a case manager to deliver care and liaise between the GP, specialist, and client [2]. It is a complex intervention which contains many essential elements, although it may be impossible to identify any one active element [3]. Usually collaborative care involves screening, education, changes in practice routines, and developments in information technology [4].

The consultation liaison model

In this model, the primary care provider (PCP) maintains a central role in the delivery of mental health care to the individual, but receives advice and support from a mental health specialist [1]. The main hypothesized outcome is therefore an improvement in PCPs' management or detection of mental health problems.

The replacement model

In this way of working, PCPs refer people with mental health problems to a mental health worker (MHW) operating within primary care, who assumes responsibility for the management of the client's problem by providing psychological or psychosocial intervention. It is hypothesized that the cost of employing a MHW, such as a psychiatrist, psychologist, or mental health nurse, will be offset by reductions in health care utilization or consultation time with primary care professionals. The MHW may also indirectly change the behavior of PCPs by raising awareness of mental health issues and management approaches [5].

General adult mental health services

Acute inpatient care

Although there is a consensus that acute inpatient services are necessary, the number of beds required is highly contingent upon which other services exist locally, and upon local social and cultural characteristics [6]. Acute inpatient care commonly absorbs most of the mental health budget [7], and therefore minimizing the use of bed days—for example by reducing the average length of stay—may be an important goal, especially if the resources released in this way can be used to pay for other service components [8–11].

Community mental health teams (CMHTs)

CMHTs, which are sometimes known in the UK as "primary care liaison teams", are the mainstay of community mental health services. The simplest model of provision of community care is for generic (nonspecialized) CMHTs to provide the full range of interventions, staffed by multidisciplinary personnel. These often prioritize adults with severe mental illness, for a local defined geographical catchment area [12–20]. The central issue here is that CMHTs can offer case management and continuity of care [21], as well as mobility. In other words, they can arrange appointments with patients at hospitals, clinics, community mental health centers, or at the patients' own homes. At the same time, it needs to be recognized that for patients not able or not willing to go to health facilities, this flexibility is necessary but not sufficient for proper care. Alongside the need for mobility is the requirement to deliver *effective* treatment when clinical encounters do take place [22].

Long-term community-based residential care

This type of care is necessary for those who need help to manage self-care and other aspects of daily living [23]. In medium- and high-income settings, when patients who have previously received long-term inpatient care for many years are discharged to community care, the outcomes are favorable for the majority [24] (the evidence for low-income settings is not clear). Nevertheless, the range and capacity of community-based residential long-term care that will be needed in any particular area is also highly dependent upon which other services are available locally, and upon social and cultural factors, such as the amount of family care that is available [25].

Outpatient/ambulatory clinics

This has been described as "office-based practice which aims to provide support and maintenance therapy for people with mental disorders" [26]. Care may be delivered by a medical practitioner, psychiatrist, or specialized nurse, who may assess symptoms, identify adverse effects, adjust medication, assist with social problems, and deliver therapy. Although there is surprisingly little evidence on the effectiveness of outpatient clinic care [27], there is a strong clinical consensus in many countries that this is a relatively efficient way to organize the provision of assessment and treatment, providing that the clinic sites are accessible to local populations. Nevertheless, these clinics are simply methods of arranging clinical contact between staff and patients, and so the key issue is the *content* of the clinical interventions, namely the delivery of treatments that are evidence-based [28–30].

Work and occupation

Rates of unemployment among people with mental disorders are usually much higher than in the general population [31]. Traditional methods of occupation have not been shown to be effective in leading to open-market employment [32–34]. For areas with medium levels of resources it is reasonable at this stage to make pragmatic decisions about the provision of work and day-care services, especially based upon the priorities and preferences of the patient/service user and carer/family member groups concerned [35], which will increasingly focus upon the importance of personal recovery [36]. At the same time, it may be relevant to take into account the accumulating evidence for supported employment models (see below) [37, 38].

Specialized services

Alternatives to acute inpatient care

* *Acute day hospitals:* These are facilities which offer programs of day treatment for those with acute and severe psychiatric problems, as an alternative to admission to inpatient units. Data from national surveys in Germany, England, Poland, Slovakia, and the Czech Republic, during 2001 and 2002, indicate that there is no consistent model of care [39].
* *Crisis houses:* These are houses in community settings which are staffed by trained mental health professionals and offer admission for some patients who would otherwise be admitted to hospital. A wide variety of respite houses, havens, and refuges have been developed, but "crisis house" is used here to mean a facility that is an alternative to noncompulsory hospital admission.
* *Home-treatment/crisis-resolution teams:* These are mobile community mental health teams offering assessment for patients in psychiatric crises, and providing intensive treatment and care at home [40].

Specialized community mental health teams (CMHTs)

* *Assertive community treatment (ACT):* This is a specialized mobile outreach treatment for those with severe and persistent mental disorders who have a history of high resource use, complex needs, and difficulty in maintaining engagement with services. It is a well-defined approach in which the full range of care is provided to a small, shared caseload by a

specialist, multidisciplinary team. The emphasis is on continuity of care, maintaining contact with service users, and building relationships [41].

- *Early-intervention teams:* The rationale for this service is that increased intervention in the early stages of psychosis or for people with prodromal symptoms may lead to improved outcomes. Early intervention for psychosis involves two distinct elements: early detection and phase-specific treatment [42].

Alternative types of long-stay community residential care

These are usually replacements for long-stay wards in psychiatric institutions [43–45]. Three main categories of such residential care can be identified:

- *24-hour staffed residential care:* This may include high-staffed hostels, residential care homes, or nursing homes, depending on whether the staff have professional qualifications. These facilities aim to maximize the social functioning and independence of the patient while optimizing medication and psychosocial interventions [23].
- *Day-staffed residential facilities:* These are hostels or residential homes which are staffed during the day.
- *Lower supported accommodation:* These are minimally supported hostels or residential homes with visiting staff.

Specialized outpatient/ambulatory clinics

These provide office-based, specialist-delivered treatment to specific groups, such as those with eating disorders, dual diagnosis, post-traumatic stress disorder, or treatment-resistant affective or psychotic disorders, as well as mentally ill mothers with babies and mentally disordered offenders. They may also deliver specialized forms of psychotherapy, for instance cognitive-behavioral therapy (CBT). Local decisions about whether to establish such specialist clinics will depend upon several factors, including their relative priority in relation to the other specialist services described, identified service gaps, and the financial opportunities available [27].

Specialized forms of work and occupation

These help mentally ill people find work, as unemployment rates in this group are high. In many high-income settings rates of unemployment among people with severe mental illness exceed 90% [46, 47]. Consumer and carer advocacy groups usually set work/occupation as one of their highest priorities, to enhance both functional status and quality of life [48, 49]. Services may offer a period of training before trying to place clients in open employment (pre-vocational training), or may place clients in competitive employment whilst providing on-the-job support (supported employment) [50]. Supported employment services are intended to be integrated within community mental health services and to be based on client preferences.

References

[1] Bower PJ, Gilbody S. Managing common mental heatlh disorders in primary care: Conceptual models and evidence base. British Medical Journal 2005;330: 839–42.

[2] Richards DA, Lovell K, Gilbody S, Gask L, Torgerson D, Barkham M, et al. Collaborative care for depression in UK primary care: A randomized controlled trial. Psychol Med 2008;38(2):279–87.

[3] Medical Research Council. A framework for development and evaluation of RCTs for complex interventions to improve health. Medical Research Council; 2000.

[4] Fletcher J, Bower PJ, Gilbody S, Lovell K, Richards D, Gask L. Collaborative care for depression and anxiety problems in primary care (Protocol). Cochrane Database of Systematic Reviews 2007;(2):CD006525.

[5] Harkness EF, Bower PJ. On-site mental health workers delivering psychological therapy and psychosocial interventions to patients in primary care: effects on the professional practice of primary care providers. (Update of Cochrane Database Syst Rev 2000;(3):CD000532; PMID: 10908476). Cochrane Database Syst Rev 2009;(1):CD000532.

[6] Thornicroft G, Tansella M. The Mental Health Matrix: A Manual to Improve Services. Cambridge: Cambridge University Press; 1999.

[7] Knapp M, Chisholm D, Astin J, Lelliott P, Audini B. The cost consequences of changing the hospital–community balance: The mental health residential care study. Psychol Med 1997;27(3):681–92.

[8] Lasalvia A, Tansella M. Acute in-patient care in modern, community-based mental health servi where and how? Epidemiol Psichiatr Soc 2010;19(4):275–81.

[9] Totman J, Mann F, Johnson S. Is locating acute wards in the general hospital an essential element in psychiatric reform? The UK experience. Epidemiol Psichiatr Soc 2010;19(4):282–6.

[10] Sederer LI. Inpatient psychiatry: Why do we need it? Epidemiol Psichiatr Soc 2010;19(4):291–5.

[11] Lelliott P, Bleksley S. Improving the quality of acute inpatient care. Epidemiol Psichiatr Soc 2010;19(4):287–90.

[12] Thornicroft G, Becker T, Holloway F, Johnson S, Leese M, McCrone P, et al. Community mental health teams: Evidence or belief? Br J Psychiatry 1999;175: 508–13.

[13] Department of Health. Community Mental Health Teams, Policy Implementation Guidance. London: Department of Health; 2002.

[14] Tyrer P, Morgan J, Van Horn E, Jayakody M, Evans K, Brummell R, et al. A randomised controlled study of close monitoring of vulnerable psychiatric patients. Lancet 1995;345(8952):756–9.

[15] Tyrer P, Evans K, Gandhi N, Lamont A, Harrison-Read P, Johnson T. Randomised controlled trial of two models of care for discharged psychiatric patients. BMJ 1998;316(7125):106–9.

[16] Thornicroft G, Wykes T, Holloway F, Johnson S, Szmukler G. From efficacy to effectiveness in community mental health services. PRiSM Psychosis Study. Br J Psychiatry 1998;173:423–7.

[17] Simmonds S, Coid J, Joseph P, Marriott S, Tyrer P. Community mental health team management in severe mental illness: A systematic review. Br J Psychiatry 2001;178:497–502.

[18] Tyrer S, Coid J, Simmonds S, Joseph P, Marriott S. Community mental health teams (CMHTs) for people with severe mental illnesses and disordered personality. Cochrane Review. Oxford: Update Software; 2003.

[19] Burns T. Generic versus specialist mental health teams. In: Thornicroft G, Szmukler G, editors. Textbook of Community Psychiatry. Oxford: Oxford University Press; 2001. pp. 231–41.

[20] Sytema S, Micciolo R, Tansella M. Continuity of care for patients with schizophrenia and related disorders: A comparative south-Verona and Groningen case-register study. Psychol Med 1997;27(6):1355–62.

[21] Dieterich M, Irving CB, Park B, Marshall M. Intensive case management for severe mental illness. Cochrane Database Syst Rev 2010;(10):CD007906.

[22] Malone D, Newron-Howes G, Simmonds S, Marriot S, Tyrer P. Community mental health teams (CMHTs) for people with severe mental illnesses and disordered personality. (Update of Cochrane Database Syst Rev 2000;(2):CD000270; PMID: 10796336). Cochrane Database of Systematic Reviews 2007;(3):CD000270.

[23] Macpherson R, Edwards TR, Chilvers R, David C, Elliott HJ. Twenty-four hour care for schizophrenia. Cochrane Database Syst Rev 2009;(2):CD004409.

[24] Shepherd G, Macpherson R. Residential care. In: Thornicroft G, Szmukler GI, Mueser KT, Drake RE, editors. Oxford Textbook of Community Mental Health. Oxford: Oxford University Press; 2011. pp. 232–44.

[25] van Wijngaarden GK, Schene A, Koeter M, Becker T, Knudsen HC, Tansella M, et al. People with schizophrenia in five European countries: Conceptual similarities and intercultural differences in family caregiving. Schizophr Bull 2003;29(3): 573–86.

[26] Shek E, Stein AT, Shansis FM, Marshall M, Crowther R, Tyrer P. Day hospital versus out-patient care for people with schizophrenia. Cochrane Database Syst Rev 2009;(4):CD003240.

[27] Becker T, Koesters M. Psychiatric outpatient clinics. In: Thornicroft G, Szmukler GI, Mueser KT, Drake RE, editors. Oxford Textbook of Community Mental Health. Oxford: Oxford University Press; 2011. pp. 179–91.

[28] Nathan P, Gorman J. A Guide to Treatments that Work, 2nd ed. Oxford: Oxford University Press; 2002.

[29] Roth A, Fonagy P. What Works for Whom? A Critical Review of Psychotherapy Research. New York: Guildford Press; 1996.

[30] BMJ Books. Clinical Evidence, volume 9. London: BMJ Books; 2003.

[31] Warner R. Recovery from Schizophrenia: Psychiatry and Political Economy. Hove: Brunner-Routledge; 2004.

[32] Shepherd G. Theory and Practice of Psychiatric Rehabilitation. Chichester: Wiley; 1990.

[33] Rosen A, Barfoot K. Day care and occupation: Structured rehabilitation and recovery programmes and work. In: Thornicroft G, Szmukler G, editors. Textbook of Community Psychiatry. Oxford: Oxford University Press; 2001. pp. 296–308.

[34] Marshall M, Crowther R, Almaraz-Serrano A, Creed F, Sledge W, Kluiter H, et al. Systematic reviews of the effectiveness of day care for people with severe

mental disorders: (1) Acute day hospital versus admission; (2) Vocational rehabilitation; (3) Day hospital versus outpatient care. Health Technol.Assess. 2001;5(21): 1–75.

[35] Cleary M, Freeman A, Walter G. Carer participation in mental health service delivery. International Journal of Mental Health Nursing 2006;15(3):189–94.

[36] Slade M. Personal recovery and mental illness. A guide for mental health professionals. Cambridge: Cambridge University Press; 2009.

[37] Catty J, Burns T, Comas A. Day centres for severe mental illness. Cochrane Review. The Cochrane Library, Issue 1. Oxford: Update Software; 2003.

[38] Becker DR, Bond GR, Drake RE. Individual placement and support: The evidence-based practice of supported employment. In: Thornicroft G, Szmukler GI, Mueser KT, Drake RE, editors. Oxford Textbook of Community Mental Health. Oxford: Oxford University Press; 2011. pp. 204–17.

[39] Kallert TW, Glockner M, Priebe S, Briscoe J, Rymaszewska J, Adamowski T, et al. A comparison of psychiatric day hospitals in five European countries: Implications of their diversity for day hospital research. Social Psychiatry & Psychiatric Epidemiology 2004;39(10):777–88.

[40] Johnson S, Needle J, Bindman J, Thornicroft G. Crisis Resolution and Home Treatment in Mental Health. Cambridge: Cambridge University Press; 2008.

[41] Department of Health. Mental Health Policy Implementation Guide. Department of Health; 2001.

[42] Marshall M, Lockwood A. Early Intervention for psychosis. (Update in Cochrane Database Syst Rev 2006;(4):CD004718; PMID: 17054213). Cochrane Database Syst Rev 2004;(2):CD004718.

[43] Shepherd G, Muijen M, Dean R, Cooney M. Residential care in hospital and in the community—Quality of care and quality of life. Br J Psychiatry 1996;168(4): 448–56.

[44] Shepherd G, Murray A. Residential care. In: Thornicroft G, Szmukler G, editors. Textbook of Community Psychiatry. Oxford: Oxford University Press; 2001. pp. 309–20.

[45] Trieman N, Smith HE, Kendal R, Leff J. The TAPS Project 41: Homes for life? Residential stability five years after hospital discharge. Team for the Assessment of Psychiatric Services. Community Ment Health J 1998;34(4):407–17.

[46] Thornicroft G, Tansella M, Becker T, Knapp M, Leese M, Schene A, et al. The Personal Impact of Schizophrenia in Europe. Schizophrenia Research 2004;69:125–32.

[47] Marwaha S, Johnson S, Bebbington P, Stafford M, Angermeyer MC, Brugha T, et al. Rates and correlates of employment in people with schizophrenia in the UK, France and Germany. British Journal of Psychiatry 2007;191:30–7.

[48] Thornicroft G, Rose D, Huxley P, Dale G, Wykes T. What are the research priorities of mental health service users? Journal of Mental Health 2002;11:1–5.

[49] Becker DR, Drake RE, Farabaugh A, Bond GR. Job preferences of clients with severe psychiatric disorders participating in supported employment programs. Psychiatr Serv 1996;47(11):1223–6.

[50] Marshall M, Bond C, Huxley P. Vocational rehabilitation for people with severe mental illness. Cochrane Database Syst Rev 2001;(2):CD003080.

Questions from a survey conducted with regional experts in the Africa region

1 Do you have a policy/strategy for implementation of community mental health services in your country? If no, have there been any smaller-scale attempts to develop community mental health services?

    A Please describe the components of community mental health care that are present in your country.

    B Do you have mental health services outside of a hospital setting (in-patient or outpatient)?

    C How do community mental health services link with primary care services?

    D Are all primary care workers trained in mental health care, or just selected workers?

    E What kinds of personnel are present in community mental health services?

    F How much mental health training have the personnel received?

    G How far do people have to travel from their homes in order to obtain mental health care?

    H How much of the country is covered by community mental health services?

2 How would you define community-oriented mental health care in your setting?

3 In developing community mental health services, what were you aiming for? What benefits did you hope for?

4 What progress has been made towards achieving aims?

5 How did you manage to achieve what you did?

Community Mental Health: putting policy into practice globally, First Edition. Graham Thornicroft, Maya Semrau, Atalay Alem, Robert E. Drake, Hiroto Ito, Jair Mari, Peter McGeorge, and R. Thara. © 2011 John Wiley & Sons, Ltd. Published 2011 by John Wiley & Sons, Ltd.

6 What are the challenges you faced on the way? (As many as you can identify.) How did you overcome them? What advice would you have for others?
7 What have you learnt?
8 Have you formally evaluated the service in any way? If so, could we have a copy of the report/publication?
9 Do you know of anybody else we should speak to?

APPENDIX C
Internet resources

Global Web sites

World Health Organization: http://www.who.int/en
The World Bank: http://www.worldbank.org
The Global Programme to Fight the Stigma and Discrimination because of Schizophrenia of the World Psychiatric Association (WPA): http://www.openthedoors.com
Principles for the Protection of Persons with Mental Illness and the Improvement of Mental Health Care. Resolution Adopted by General Assembly of the United Nations 46/119 of 17 December 1991: http://www.unhchr.ch/html/menu3/b/68.htm

Web sites for the Africa region

Mental Health and Poverty Project:
http://workhorse.pry.uct.ac.za:8080/MHAPP
Africa Regional Centre for WHO: www.afro.who.int

Web sites for the Australasia and South Pacific region

Beyondblue (NGO working to address issues associated with depression, anxiety, and related substance-misuse disorders): http://www.beyondblue.org.au
The Black Dog Institute (clinical, research, and educational body dedicated to improving understanding, diagnosis and treatment of depression and bipolar disorder): http://www.blackdoginstitute.org.au

Web sites for the Europe region

WHO Regional Office for Europe: http://www.euro.who.int/en/home
WHO European Health For All Database:
http://data.euro.who.int/hfadb

Community Mental Health: putting policy into practice globally, First Edition. Graham Thornicroft, Maya Semrau, Atalay Alem, Robert E. Drake, Hiroto Ito, Jair Mari, Peter McGeorge, and R. Thara. © 2011 John Wiley & Sons, Ltd. Published 2011 by John Wiley & Sons, Ltd.

National Institute for Health and Clinical Excellence (NICE) (UK):
http://www.nice.org.uk

The Changing Minds campaign of the Royal College of Psychiatrists:
http://www.rcpsych.ac.uk/campaigns/cminds

UK Disability Rights Commission: http://www.drc-gb.org

Evidence of effective interventions against stigma, from research conducted at the Institute of Psychiatry, King's College London: http://
www.iop.kcl.ac.uk/iopweb/departments/home/default.aspx?locator=
461

The Mental Disability Advocacy Center: http://www.mdac.info

Disability Rights International: http://www.disabilityrightsintl.org

Rethink and the Institute of Psychiatry, King's College London (source
of evidence-based information on a range of mental illnesses):
http://www.mentalhealthcare.org.uk

The "See Me" campaign (challenges stigma and discrimination around
mental ill-health in Scotland): http://www.seemescotland.org

"Shift" (initiative of the National Institute for Mental Health in England (NIMHE), to tackle stigma and discrimination surrounding mental health issues): http://www.shift.org.uk

Web sites for the North America region

US Department of Health and Human Services Resource Center to Address Discrimination and Stigma: http://www.adscenter.org

The Bazelon Center for Mental Health Law: http://www.bazelon.org

The Chicago Consortium for Stigma Research:
http://www.stigmaresearch.org

The National Empowerment Center: http://www.power2u.org

The National Stigma Clearinghouse: http://community2.webtv.net/
stigmanet/AbouttheNational/index.html

University of Hartford's resource page on fighting discrimination and
stigma: http://uhaweb.hartford.edu/owahl/resources.htm

Web sites for the Latin America and
Caribbean region

Página da União Européia sobre saúde na América Latina:
http://www.healthinlatinamerica.org

Oganização Panamericana de saúde: http://www.paho.org

Associação Psiquiátrica da América Latina http://www.apalweb.org

Ministério da Saúde do Brasil: http://www.saude.gov.br

Ministério da Saúde de Cuba: http://www.sld.cu

Ministério da Saúde da Costa Rica: http://www.ministeriodesalud.go.cr

Ministério da Saúde da Venezuela: http://www.msds.gov.ve

Ministério da Saúde do Peru: http://www.minsa.gob.pe

Ministério da Saúde da Bolívia: http://www.sns.gov.bo

Ministério da Saúde da Argentina: http://www.msal.gov.ar

Ministério da Saúde do Panamá: http://www.minsa.gob.pa

Ministério da Saúde do Chile: http://www.minsal.cl

Associação Brasileira de Psiquiatria: http://www.abpbrasil.org.br

Associação Peruana de Psiquiatria: http://www.app.org.pe

Associação Mexicana de Psiquiatria: http://www.psiquiatrasapm.org.mx

Associação Porto-Riquenha de Psiquiatria:
  http://www.puertoricopsychiatricsociety.org

Associação Argentina de Psiquiatras: http://www.aap.org.ar

Sociedade de Psiquiatria do Uruguai: http://www.spu.org.uy

Sociedade de Neurologia, Psiquiatria e Neurocirurgia do Chile:
  http://www.sonepsyn.cl

Sociedade de Psiquiatria da Venezuela: http://www.svp.org.ve

Index

Community Mental Health: putting policy into practice globally, First Edition. Graham Thornicroft,
Maya Semrau, Atalay Alem, Robert E. Drake, Hiroto Ito, Jair Mari, Peter McGeorge, and R. Thara.
© 2011 John Wiley & Sons, Ltd. Published 2011 by John Wiley & Sons, Ltd.